# Is this really happening?

To Aunt J.

With Love

Jewell

x

# Is this really happening?

Maria  de la Mann

easyBroom

Is this really happening?

An easyBroom book

Copyright © 2022 Maria de la Mann

ISBN 978-0957628861

The right of Maria de la Mann to be identified as the author of this work has been asserted in accordance with sections 77 and 78 of the Copyright, Designs and Patents Act 1988

Cover painting and cover design: Maria de la Mann

A catalogue record of this book is available from
The British Library

## Books by the author

Verity Red's Diary (A story of surviving M.E.)

Love & Best Witches

Verity Writes Again

Verity Red (part one)

Verity Red (part two)

Verity Red (part three)

*for Jim & Pauline Logan*

*Dedicated to the memory of*

*Patricia Anstey, my little brother Peter
and dear old dad*

# Acknowledgements

A whole book full of thank yous to my partner Nigel for doing a wonderful job, helping me put *another* book together. And to his dear sister Julia for beautifully proof reading *another* book.

To my cats Diamanda and Lovely, for making me smile and laugh every day, especially when they sit on my notes or tread on my laptop keys to improve my writing.

Last but not least, to my favourite poets Jim Logan and his little grandson Eddie, for their delightful poems that, like my cats, make me smile and laugh.

# Prologue

Verity Red is back.

Why is she staring out of her bedroom window and wondering – Is this really happening?

Why is she trapped in a cold, pitch dark room, with a voice in her head saying – Is this really happening?

Why is she sitting in a dirty, depressing, uninhabited house and saying to herself – Is this really happening?

Why is she watching the news and thinking –

Read on....

# November

## Monday 5th

9.00 a.m.    *CRASH! CRASH! CRASH!... Rumble..... Rumble..... Rumble.... CRACK!! CLUNK!!..... Clank..... Clunk... Clank... CRUNCH!* Clitter, clatter, clitter, clatter of caterpillar tracks – *right outside* our *ruddy* house!

9.01 a.m.    There's an angry man stomping around in the muddy gravel. Sweating... Swearing... Shouting. His ruddy red complexion under a white hard hat.

9.02 a.m.    Our house is shaking. Like me on a frosty morning, plodding to the bird table, without my soft, woolly bobble hat protecting me from the ruddy cold weather.

9.03 a.m.    The Victorian houses in our little street are trembling with fear. They are *very frightened*. TV aerials on rooftops sway at angles, like fur on a threatened cat.

9.04 a.m.    The demolition monsters have arrived to demolish the car park, car showroom and community hall, opposite where we live. We knew they would appear one day. We were warned. But we shut it out of our minds. Closed the door to the memory of *that letter*. And locked it. Securely.

9.05 a.m.    But now the door has been flung wide open, a nasty freezing draught has flown in, chilled us to the bone, *and* it's impossible to ignore the inevitable – as our windows rattle, the floor boards shake, and cans of paint rattle in the cellar.

9.06 a.m.    The surface of my cup of tea quivers. Or maybe I should say the meniscus quivers. I like the word

1

meniscus. The meniscus in the circumference of my cuppa quivers. I like the word circumference too.

9.07 a.m.     Mmm.... *meniscuss*.... *circummference*.... Mmm.... my mind is swaying at all angles, like the TV aerials – with all the noise and disruption.

9.08 a.m.     Now the meniscus in my cuppa is sloshing about like a miniature stormy sea. A storm in a teacup!

9.09 a.m.     I am not laughing.

9.10 a.m.     The cats in our neighbourhood must think we are experiencing earthquakes. They will be pussy-footing around their territory full of feline fear.

9.11 a.m.     There's a JCB that's *so close* at times. *SO HORRI-BLY CLOSE* – one swing of the monster's long neck in the wrong direction, and the big head (with lots of teeth) could come crashing through our bedroom window. Well, if the neck was *very* stretched out, it would. Or, if maybe the driver of the metal monster returned from a lunchtime drink at our local watering hole (worse for wear), then lost control of his pedals and levers, it could be disastrous – these things *do happen.*

* * * * * * * *

10.00 a.m.    I'm still sitting on the bed, staring out of the bed-room window watching metal jaws plunging into dark gloom-grey tarmac. Gouging. Ripping. Destroying. Tearing-up the once-was-a-car-park in our once-was-a-peaceful street, like marzipan peeled off a fruit cake, strip by strip – then thrown aside onto the floor.

10.03 a.m.  Our peaceful little street is peaceful no more.

10.04 a.m.  I need comfort food.

10.07 a.m.  In kitchen.

10.08 a.m.  My M.E. diet is mentally thrown aside into the bin.

10.09 a.m.  I fancy a nice slice of fruit cake. Without the marzipan.

10.10 a.m.  Make mental note to put fruit cake on shopping list.

10.11 a.m.  I will feel much more peaceful, full of fruit cake.

\* \* \* \* \* \* \* \* \*

2.30 p.m.  After watching *Loose Women* (Nadine and her team of celebs digging for gossip from other celebs) and *Time Team* (Tony and his team of archaeologists digging in the hope of finding a Roman burial ground), I rested my eyes from the TV screen, sitting on the bed once more, staring out of the window. Quietly observing.

2.31 p.m.  Unlike Nadine and her team of chatty ladies, digging for gossip with laughter. Or Tony's team of weathered archaeologists, cheerfully digging, then painstakingly scraping away at a skull (a femur here, a fibula there), then *ever so gently* and reverently removing their finds – workmen miserably stomped around shouting in the cold, or drove the metal monsters to destruction – mercilessly ripping out railings and wooden fencing. *Rip... Tear... Crash... Rip... Tare... Crash...* The metal monsters *hell-bent* on destruction. Or maybe I should say, *metal-bent*.

3

2.32 p.m.   I am not smiling.

2.33 p.m.   Diamanda is sitting in the bedroom window, watching the world in a cat-like way. Cats are *such experts* at just sitting. And watching. I have learned a lot from my cats over the years. How to be contented to just *sit*. Not move for *quite a while*. And just watch. Although I haven't mastered the art of getting excited about a long piece of string or an empty cardboard box... I'm working on it.

2.34 p.m.   Diamanda's long black tail twitches from side to side. Her ears are a little flattened – what I call owl ears. They show she *does not approve at all* of the horrible loud noises, all the dreadful unsettling racket. And the house shaking *so much*, she feels that the walls may crumble and fall down around her ears and whiskers at any moment. This is all *most disagreeable.*

She sniffs – little black nose in the air.

2.35 p.m.   I smile.

2.36 p.m.   Recalling my tabby cat, from many moons ago. She had owl ears when I sang or played my guitar. This was *most understandable.*

2.37 p.m.   I gently stroke Diamanda's silky black head, making comforting noises.

2.38 p.m.   I kiss her front paws – black with white diamond-shaped markings.

2.39 p.m.   She softly purrs.

2.40 p.m.     Ears returned to contented-cat-position.

* * * * * * * *

3.00 p.m.

ME:     Is this really happening? (pointing towards the car park).

BEN:     Yeah (looking grim).

ME:     We knew it would one day didn't we, even before we were informed by post.

BEN:     Yeah.

ME:     Just what you need isn't it, *another* noisy housing estate nearby, when you've *only just* retired. Well, semi-retired. And you've been really, *really* lookin' forward to a more peaceful, less stressful life for years, away from noisy office life. Writing music, playing your guitar or practising for digs in pubs.

BEN:     You mean gigs in pubs (picking up guitar).

ME:     Oh yes.... but I *do dig* your music! So does Diamanda, she doesn't flatten her ears like an owl when you play.

BEN:     Yeah (grinning)...... I'm poppin' to Sainsbury's later, want anything?

ME:     I'd love a small fruit cake.

BEN:     You *are* a small fruit cake dear.

* * * * * * * *

4.35 p.m.

ME: The noise and house shaking has *finally* stopped. Peace at last.

BEN: Yeah (handing me a slice of fruit cake on a plate).

ME: Ah, thank you. A *piece* at last.

* * * * * * * *

5.05 p.m. POP! POP! *BANG! BANG! BANG! BOOOOOOOM!*

5.06 p.m. Diamanda hides behind the sofa.

5.07 p.m. *WHIZZZZZZ! Whoooosh! Whoooosh! Wheeeeee!*

5.08 p.m. *CRACKLE! CRACKLE! CRACKLE! BANG!..... Phut! Phut!....* CRACK! CRACK!

5.09 p.m. In the distance – *Crickle! Crackle! WHOOOSH..... POW!...... POW!........ POW!......* **BANG!**

ME: I forgot it was bonfire night.

BEN: So did I (putting on headphones).

## Tuesday 6th

10.05 a.m. It's eerily quiet in the car park today. Huge piles of rubble are dotted here and there. No workmen in sight on site. The metal monsters are motionless; their necks, arms and claws tucked in like sleeping cats.

10.06 a.m. Diamanda dozes in the bedroom window, tail tucked in neatly, peacefully purring. I perch on the bed sleepily surveying the destruction.

10.07 a.m.   I notice a large pile of wooden fence posts. They would have made a brilliant bonfire for last night's celebrations. The workmen could have made a fantastic fiery blaze after work, and warmed themselves up. Maybe baked some jacket potatoes in the heart of the fire, then set off a few fireworks. I could have enjoyed them from my window.

10.08 a.m.   It would have been a small compensation for all the disruption. The silly workmen didn't think of that, did they. No. *Most disappointing!*

10.10 a.m.   Two big black crows, who usually peck for bugs (or whatever they can lay their beaks on) in the car park, strut about on a pile of rubble. They bring to mind portly old gentlemen, wearing black suits (arms behind their backs) gravely checking-out the situation.

10.14 a.m.   Ooh, something is happening. There's a rumbling noise. Something has come to life. The monsters must have woken up. There's a black one at the far end of the car park, I hadn't noticed it before. Its yellow eyes are flashing brightly.

10.15 a.m.   I can't see clearly what's going on, piles of rubble are in the way. *Most frustrating!*

10.16 a.m.   Hmm, something else is occurring. Two workmen have appeared, the crows fly off, squawking disapproval. The men are chatting. I can't hear what they are saying, so I can't be nosey. Bored now.

10.17 a.m.  I lie down on the bed. Plonk. Like an egg in flour. I will not be beaten. I will survive this.

10.18 a.m.  Recalling the small crowd of people I saw in the car park (that's more a building site now) the other day, wearing yellow hard hats and matching waistcoats, standing around in the sunshine. Some of the crowd were women, and when a man began to speak and they all gathered around to listen, I supposed they were the planning department having a meeting. There were twenty-five of them. I counted. Something to do. A small achievement for the day. A little observation to exercise my tired old brain.

10.19 a.m.  The gathering brought to mind a menacing cluster of shiny yellow insects, planning a spot of crop devastation. I must have been having a bad day. On a good day, I would have imagined a cluster of shiny yellow buttercups, glistening in the sunshine, swaying gently in the breeze.

10.30 a.m.  I sit up to see if anything interesting is happening yet. Yes! The two workmen are flapping their arms at each other, looking disgruntled. Unlike the crows, they are not about to fly away – will there be a fight?!

10.31 a.m.  Shall I call the police if they start beating each other with their hard hats?

10.32 a.m.  One of the men is on his mobile phone, pacing about at a distance from the other man.

10.35 a.m.  Ooh, another workman has appeared with a length of orange hose pipe, but they are all disappearing from my view now. Drat. It was just getting interesting.

10.36 a.m.   It is starting to rain.

10.37 a.m.   I watch the rain trickling down the window pane. I expect soon the car park will be full of muddy puddles and disgruntled workmen splashing about.

11.00 a.m.   Perusing TV Weekly.

11.01 a.m.   Fortunately I've got Tony and his team of archaeologists to look forward to at midday. They will be searching for the remains of an Iron Age fort today. Then examining mosaic pieces in a Cotswold field. Great – will go down well with a nice cuppa and slice of fruit cake.

11.03 a.m.   Notice there's a new series starting: *When Demolitions Go Wrong* – Most demolitions go off without a hitch, but sometimes disaster strikes, devastating other properties, and injuring or even killing innocent spectators. This documentary uses first-hand testimony to retell the stories behind demolition disasters. I will not watch – give me nightmares.

* * * * * * * *

1.25 p.m.   *Crash!... Crash!... Crash!... Crash!* A JCB is digging an *enormous* hole. Fortunately this is happening on TV – looks like an episode of *Columbo*. The detective is standing, wearing a grey raincoat, peering down the hole on a building site, mopping his brow, with a *most-concerned-weathered-worried* expression – no doubt expecting to see something gruesome, like a dead body, with just the head sticking out.

1.26 p.m.   I notice the workmen in *Columbo* are wearing white, yellow, blue and green hard hats, but no bright waist-

coats. I guess in 1970's America, workmen on building sites were not issued with bright waistcoats –
the variety of colourful hard hats made up for it
though.

1.30 p.m.    Ben joins me in the sitting room.

BEN:    *Columbo?*

ME:    Yes.

BEN:    The building site in this looks like the *lovely view*
opposite our house.

ME:    Mm, but with more colourful hard hats bobbing
about.

BEN:    Yeah.

ME:    I used to work in a planning department with a
man whose initials were JCB – I saw them on his
drawings.

BEN:    Was he a big muscly man?

ME:    Yes! Guess what his name was?

BEN:    John something?

ME:    No, guess again.

BEN:    Must I?

ME:    Yes, *Columbo* is boring.

BEN:    Joshua? Jack?

ME:        No.

BEN:       Jake? James?

ME:        Correct, James! Now guess his second name.

BEN:       Colin? Chris?

ME:        No.

BEN:       Clive? Carl?

ME:        Nope.

BEN:       I give up. Can't wait for you to tell me.

ME:        James Cedric Buchanan. Sounds posh doesn't it.

BEN:       Was he?

ME:        No.

BEN:       Well, I'm glad we've got that sorted. I can rest easy in my bed tonight.

## Wednesday 7th

11.00 a.m.   *OH NO!! PANIC! Oh God!* Diamanda has wandered onto the building site, *right in front* of a JCB, and a pile of rubble has started to fall dangerously close to her head.

11.01 a.m.   I'm running out of the front door in my pyjamas and dressing gown, around the corner and out of our street, in search of the entrance to the building site.

11.02 a.m.　A crowd of people are visiting the site. It's a royal visit. Princess Eugenie and her new husband Jack, Prince William and Kate (with her new hairstyle), Prince Harry and Megan (with her new baby bump) stand, smiling and peering into an enormous hole in the ground.

11.03 a.m.　They all laugh as I run to Diamanda, scoop her up in my arms, and a pile of rubble from the jaws of a JCB starts to fall near my head. Then Columbo appears, looking deeply concerned.

11.04 a.m.　Yes. *It was all a dream.*

11.05 a.m.　Diamanda treads on my head and wakes me up from a late morning nap on the sofa. Celebrity Weekly is lying on my chest – Prince Harry and Megan smile out of the front cover.

11.06 a.m.　*Crash! Crunch! Crash! Crunch! Rumble..... rumble.* The house is shaking so much at times, the pictures in the clip frames on our walls are rattling.

11.15 a.m.　I'm in the kitchen, and I can't believe the saucepans on the cooker are rattling madly every time there's a particularly big rumble – I have to laugh.

11.20 a.m.　Ben returns from a trip to Sainsbury's with bulging carrier bags and starts to unpack the shopping. I help with the light things.

11.22 a.m.　I plod upstairs with a tube of toothpaste and four toilet rolls. In the bathroom the leaves on my plants are trembling, and I imagine the water in the toilet is quivering too, but I don't bother to investigate – the toilet needs a clean and I haven't got the energy at the moment.

* * * * * * * *

1.00 pm.

ME: The monsters with big-toothed-jaws and claws, are grazing on the tarmac in the car park. And a black skip has appeared, maybe it's a watering trough for the monsters.

BEN: I'm sure it is dear. It's been raining so heavily they'll be able to enjoy a nice long drink. And I see the car showroom has been completely demolished now.

ME: Yes. *Completely demolished.* That's exactly how I feel (big sigh) after all the de-cluttering we've been doing lately.

BEN: You need to pace yourself more.

ME: *I know.* But it's *so hard* when you're feeling stressed because you've recently lost a beloved pet, and *really need* to do something to take your mind off how *madly sad* you feel. And you want to move house NOW, because you *can't stand* your noisy neighbours and the lovely view you've had for twenty-something years is going to be replaced with a housing estate, *and* you need a view because you spend SO MUCH of your day looking out of the window when your eyes are too tired to watch TV or read or write a letter, AND you are suddenly aware that you have become a hoarder and your partner is a hoarder too. There's *so much to do* and you need *to do so much to the house* to make it sellable, and you haven't got the energy to even *think* about everything that needs to be thought about, let alone do it. *AND* you didn't realise you had quite so many books, ornaments, little keep-sakes, jigsaw puzzles, cuddly toys, candle holders, clothes, shoes, scarves, photos in frames, pictures in frames, birthday and Christmas cards (you particularly liked and kept), letters from penfriends, postcards, photographs in wallets, vinyl records, CDs, cassettes, percussion instruments and... *and.... and..... IS THIS REALLY HAPPENING?*

BEN:        I'll get you a camomile tea dear.

* * * * * * * * *

1.20 p.m.    I'm sitting on the bed, sleepily watching the little piles of rubble on the building site grow and grow, into huge mountains of broken tarmac, bricks and tree roots.

1.21 p.m.    The mountains of rubble would look far more entertaining if I placed my garden ornaments (the seven dwarves) here and there, and I could imagine them singing their digging song.

1.30 p.m.    I'm lying on the bed like a pile of rubble, singing to myself.

*We dig dig dig dig dig dig dig in our mine the whole day through*

*We dig dig dig dig dig dig dig is what we like to do*

1.31 p.m.    Diamanda does not approve of the noise coming out of my mouth – she has owl ears.

1.32 p.m.     Recall my lovely ginger cat, who passed away many moons ago. He would put his paw over my mouth when I sang. The memory makes me smile.

1.33 p.m.     Must find the energy to have a bath.

* * * * * * * *

2.05 p.m.     In bath. Luke warm water, so I don't become too drained and not be able to get out of the bath.

2.06 p.m.     Singing softly to self.

*We dig dig dig dig dig dig dig from early morn till night*

*We dig dig dig dig dig dig dig up everything in sight*

2.36 p.m.     Lying on bed, feeling nice and clean. Singing very quietly to myself, so as not to *purrturb* Diamanda. I have no energy to do the whistling bits.

*Heigh-ho, Heigh-ho*
*It's home from work we go*
*La la la la, la la la la*
*Heigh-ho, Heigh-ho*
*Heigh-ho, Heigh-ho*

3.10 p.m.     Dozing on sofa. Tony Robinson is on TV with his team of archaeologists, dig, dig, digging on *Time Team*. Today they are uncovering a Roman villa and Roman cemetery in a cornfield.

3.15 p.m.     I wonder if there will be any interesting finds when the workmen opposite our house dig deep into the building site. On *Time Team*, if they find human bones, sometimes they have to call a halt to their work while the police do an investigation – I will look out for police.

4.20 p.m.     I'm watching *90 Day Fiancé*. Sadly, it seems there are plenty of young people, gold dig, dig, digging, from foreign countries, who want to marry Americans in order to get a green card and work in the country – Women from countries like Russia, Brazil and the Ukraine. Men from Africa, Tunisia and Morocco. There's a lot of tears drip, drip, dripping on this programme. Lust is blind.

7.00 p.m.     *Coronation Street* will be good tonight. Leanne believes Nick is a changed man. But Carla is digging deep into his recent past and finds out the truth. I see trouble ahead. Lots of fireworks. *Can't wait!*

## Thursday 8th

11.25 a.m.    There's a rustling sound outside our front door. Then, *KNOCK! KNOCK! KNOCK!*

11.28 a.m.    *Hurrah!* My first Christmas parcel has arrived – small gifts and cards for family and friends, from one of my favourite catalogues.

11.29 a.m.    *Sniff.........* sniff......... *sniff.* I'm enjoying the flowery fragrances of the hand creams. Each one in a small tube that looks like an artist's paint tube. They will be perfect for artistic ladies in our family.

My nose bobs from scent to scent, like an excited bumble bee – enjoying lily of valley, honeysuckle, rose petal, lavender, white jasmine and lilac blossom.

**11.30 a.m.** *Ahh,* that gave me a buzz.

**11.32 a.m.** The Night Owl CD (late night classics) looks good – with titles like *Nectar* (I mean *Nocturn), Dreaming,* and *The Swan.* Hope dad will enjoy it.

**11.33 a.m.** The little owl on the cover is a hoot.

**11.34 a.m.** The socks make me smile. They will match the shirt I ordered for Ben – midnight blue with white music notes on staves. I will pop them in his Christmas stocking, along with the green-tinted, white chocolate sprouts (with an orangey filling) that look exactly like sprouts. Well, *almost* exactly.

**11.37 a.m.** The wildlife calendars and Christmas cards look good, better than advertised – lots of birds and bunnies, squirrels, foxes, hedgehogs, badgers and deer in the snow. Sparkly glitter on the cards. *Lots of glitter.*

**11.38 a.m.** I have silvery glitter on my hands, face and dressing gown now.

**11.40 a.m.** Starting to feel a little Christmassy all over.

* * * * * * * *

**1.20 p.m.** Watching the afternoon Christmas film on Channel 5 – *12 Gifts of Christmas.* It's a comedy about an executive who hires a personal Christmas shopper and discovers it's more about the thought than the money spent.

1.25 p.m.    Feeling a little more Christmassy.

1.30 p.m.    I wonder if mince pies are in the shops. A tasty, hot,
             fruity mince pie will make me feel *even more* Christ-
             massy. And help me resist sampling the choc sprouts
             – my body is craving sugar. And I want to stay in a
             cheerful-pre-Christmas mood, instead of a post-de-
             cluttering-of-house and really-want-to-move-house
             exhausted mood.

*  *  *  *  *  *  *  *

Our house was valued in September (and the mort-
gage is paid off), so now we have an idea of what we
can afford to buy. Ben uses a website on his Smartphone that notifies him when a property appears on
the market in our price range (in the areas we are
interested in). The wonders of modern technology!
We're looking for a bungalow near the seaside on
the Sussex or Kent coast.

There's a lot to do on the house. I can't do much,
apart from de-clutter when I have the energy, but
fortunately Ben has a friend to help him – Bill is
very handy with a paintbrush and plastering. And
we have a carpenter friend we can trust. The house
will be much more sellable when it doesn't look like
it's about to fall down, and some of the very old
carpets are replaced.

When a house pops-up that we like the look of, Ben
and his mate Bill drive to the location and take a look
from the outside. Although there's no house number
on the website (just a postcode), the houses are *fairly*
easy to find. Then Ben makes a short video on his
smartphone of the property (from the road, street or

hazardous hedgerows), and I get an idea of what the surrounding area is like. I can tell the boys enjoy making the video; they are like a couple of young lads having an adventure (like they used to when they were young), and this is especially true when, after much searching, they finally find a run-down house hidden behind a lot of undergrowth. *And* a passing neighbour tells them stories of the previous strange occupant.

It's very useful when they discover something that's not shown on a website – like the property is on a very busy main road, it's a bit of a rough area, or there's a rather undesirable looking family living in the adjoining property. SO, we know it's not worth wasting our time, or my precious energy, plodding around viewing a home and trying to imagine living there.

Sitting in the comfort of our warm home, on the sofa, watching Bill and Ben's short films with an amusing commentary, is beautifully entertaining. And *most* M.E. friendly.

4.20 p.m.

BEN: A property has come up that I think you'll really like. It's in Pevensey Bay. Detached bungalow. Bohemian.

ME: Do you like it?

BEN: Yeah.

ME: Are you going to find it with Bill?

BEN: We've already seen a house in that area – looks quiet and it's close to the beach. It's an Oyster House.

ME: Oyster House? Is it decorated with oyster shells? Did oyster fishermen live in it?

BEN: It's got a curved front, like an oyster shell. The houses were a fashionable seaside dwelling in the 1930's.

ME: *Oh lovely, can you show me the website!*

BEN: Yeah (opening laptop).

ME: Looks nice, it's got art deco-ish character. I like the long front garden and driveway. And you'd have a garage. No more hunting for a parking space. We could have little strolls on the beach. Or I could sit and watch you stroll, on one of my very tired days. This could be the home of our dreams!

BEN: Shall we view it then?

ME: *Yes let's!* I know we're not ready to sell yet, but if we *really like* a property, the chap who valued our house said we could sell ours as it is. We'll have time to do more de-cluttering and smarten up the place a bit.

BEN: I'll phone and e-mail the estate agent tomorrow.

ME: Oh goody!


## Friday 9th

2.10 p.m. *Drill….. drill….. drill.* Not on the building site, it's quiet today. Maybe they've found human bones and are waiting for the police to make an investigation.

2.11 p.m.   *Drill..... drill...... drill.* Coming from the downstairs window at the front of our house. A builder mate of Ben's is doing some repair work on the outside window ledge. Then when Ben has prepared the woodwork, his mate Bill will give the front door and window frame a lick of white paint. It will be a lot cheaper than replacing them, and help retain the cottagey feel of our house – I like the small panes of glass in the old sash window.

2.14 p.m.   Rain clouds are gathering, so Ben's mate is working as quickly as possible.

2.16 p.m.   I'm watching the comedy film, *Christmas In The Clouds,* to stay in a cheerful-pre-Christmas mood.

2.24 p.m.   During the adverts I gaze thoughtfully at our net curtains, with leaf and butterfly design. They are fairly new, fresh and white, so they won't need replacing.

3.00 p.m.   I'm enjoying the feeling of my head in the clouds – white Christmas clouds, until I'm brought down to earth with more *drill..... drill...... drilling.* Not from the building site. It's still spookily quiet. Not a hard hat in sight. Just a couple of crows plodding about, checking out the situation, nodding their heads.

3.01 p.m.   The drilling is coming from the kitchen, Ben is putting up three shelves. He meant to do this about fifteen years ago, but he never got a *round-tuit.* He said *round-tuits* were difficult to find in the shops or on the internet. And when he got around to looking for a *round-tuit,* they were out of stock. But now he has plenty of time to shop around for *round-*

*tuits,* for all the little jobs that need doing, and get the best bargain.

4.45 p.m.  *Drill...... drill...... drill.* Not from the building site or kitchen. Ben is giving a patient a filling at his dental practice. That's Ben Harper (played by actor Robert Lindsay) in the sitcom, *My Family,* with the very funny actress Zoe Wanamaker.

7.45 p.m.  *Drill...... drill...... drill.....* in *Coronation Street.* Tim attempts to drill home into Gina's deluded mind that he is still very much in love with his wife Sally (Gina's sister). Even though they've been living together happily in his house while Sally is in prison awaiting trial. Yes – they constantly have a good laugh and she's been a wonderful companion. They enjoy the same films and she makes him his favourite sandwiches for lunch. But Sally will *always* be his number one girl. And, no – he *did not* marry the wrong sister!

8.10 p.m.  *Dig..... dig..... dig.* Archive footage of old movies are dug out for the panel show, *The Imitation Game.* Contestants re-enact famous scenes from movies, provide alternative voice-overs to news footage and put unlikely words in celebrities' mouths. Entertaining, but not as good as *Coronation Street.*

8.40 p.m.  Back in *Coronation Street* it's *grill.... grill.... grill....* as Elsa grills Carla about Nick.

9.01 p.m.  In our kitchen it's *grill..... grill..... grill.* Toast and a milky drink.

9.02 p.m.  I'm looking forward to tomorrow. Will we find the home of our dreams?

9.03 p.m.    As the milk bubbles, I bubble up with excitement.

*Bubble... bubble... bubble.*

## Saturday 10th

2.00 p.m.

ME:    We're actually going to view a property! A lovely Oyster House beside the seaside. And it's a beautiful bright sunny day!

BEN:    Yes dear, best wrap up warm though, it'll be chilly near the beach. And the house will be cold, it's been empty for some time.

ME:    I'll wear me woolly hat 'n' scarf 'n' gloves. We might decide to have a look at the bay before we go home too.

BEN:    Maybe sit on the beach with a bag of chips.

ME:    I hope there will be something to sit on in the house, when I get one of my suddenly-tired-need-to-collapse-on-floor moments. I'll feel obliged to make comments like – nice sized room, needs some TLC, the bed could go there, lick of paint, sofa could go there, cosy with a new carpet. It'll be wearing.

BEN:    You or the carpet?

ME:    Very amusing dear.

BEN:    I couldn't see any furniture in the photos on the internet, the place looks unfurnished. But I explained to the estate agent that you had M.E. and would tire easily. She was very understanding because she has a friend who has M.E.

ME:     Oh, good! She won't be alarmed if I suddenly sit on the floor. And I won't have to explain myself. Let's go, I can't wait to see what could be our *dream home*. Our new world. *The world is our oyster.*

BEN:    The Oyster House could be our new world!

\* \* \* \* \* \* \* \* \*

It wasn't the dilapidated, neglected look of the outside of the place. A nice lick of paint, and it could look good as new, maybe soft seagull grey on the walls. It wasn't the grimy windows – lots of windows on the curvy bohemian front of the dwelling. After a good wash they'd let in lots of light. It wasn't the tired old terracotta pots full of dead, dried-up plants, the weeds in the driveway, unkempt lawn or weathered picket fence, with a broken gate. These things could be sorted.

It wasn't, on entry to the property, the *smell*. Or the thin urine-yellow curtains in the front room, opened in a careless way to reveal the grimy panes. The small pooh-brown Persian rug in the middle of the wooden floor. The tatty toffee-brown, seventies wooden cabinet with a broken door, in the corner. The horrible silvery lamp stand, like a misshapen Henry Moore sculpture, sitting on the cabinet. The grim, old-fashioned watercolour painting of the countryside, all mouldy greens and sick yellows, left hanging at an angle, abandoned on the grubby grey wall. These things could be replaced, and the room made to look welcoming – especially if you take Linda Barker's advice in *60 Minute Makeover*.

It wasn't the smallest, filthiest, most claustrophobic bathroom I've ever seen – like a putrid public toilet cubicle next to an old bath, with flooring that was in such a bad state of repair, it looked like it hadn't been replaced since the 1930's. Or tiles around the bath, the colour of a pale, drowned person – with the odd badly placed blue dolphin. *Or* the thought of bathing in the bath, as desirable as kissing a dead-for-days fish. OR, on *finally* opening the airing cupboard (with Ben's brut force), I thought a million huge, hairy spiders and fleas would jump out onto me – flies and poisonous insects buzzing around my head. And to open the maggot-white cupboard you had to shut yourself in the bathroom – *and* when we did, I felt I was about have a panic attack.

NO. All this was not a problem. These things could be sorted. Knock down a wall. Extend. Re-decorate. If affordable. And possible.

It wasn't the kitchen/diner. There was a wooden stool with a wobbly leg for me to perch on, resting my wobbly legs, after the shock of the bathroom. I was able to sit (while Ben chatted to the estate agent) and *admire* the tired white Formica cabinets, with round, dried-blood-red handles, like sore spots on an anaemic face. Red and white – the colours I hate most in a kitchen. But this was, as Kirsty Allsopp says on *Location, Location, Location,* just cosmetic. Although, I couldn't see what could be done about the tiny window. To see out of it, I had to lean *right* over the sink and turn my head to the right. And this made my neck hurt. And I love to be able to watch the wildlife out of my kitchen window. The squirrels and our wonderful variety of birds, make me smile every single day. SO, I decided this room could be a *right pain* in the neck.

It wasn't the corridor with raggedy old stale-orange curtains, and a frayed carpet (vaguely duck-egg-blue with bird-pooh-like stains) leading to the bedrooms. Or the small bedroom, with turquoise and purple walls, and the odd, peeling Disney sticker here and there. And a view of a neglected once-upon-a-time-white-washed brick wall, three feet from the window.

NO. We could commission Bill (a brilliant artist, as well as painter and decorator) to paint a colourful scene on the wall. Beautiful bright green rolling hills under a summers-day-blue sky, with Disney animals frolicking about – like Bambi, Goofy, Mickey Mouse, Donald Duck and Milo the lion cub.

It wasn't the not-much-bigger bedroom. I can't recall *much* about it, I must have been feeling as worn as the carpet. I just remember that, like the rest of the house, it had seen better days. I think there were dreary yellow and green walls. Stale avocado green. Dead daffodil yellow. The carpet – the painful yellows and greens of a recovering bruise. And although the room was empty, I became aware that there was a *presence* and we were unwelcome intruders. I only stayed in the room long enough to *admire* the view of the small, lumpy, neglected garden, with something dark at the end. A wall or a hedge. My memory is foggy. But gardens can be made attractive with a little imagination, hard work, and if you pay attention to Ann Maurice's advice in *House Doctor*.

It wasn't the shed, full of rusty-brown, ancient looking junk, draped with cobwebs, that didn't look safe
to enter. It could be cleared out. Or the garage. We
didn't see inside it, I don't know why. Again, I can't
remember. Maybe Ben couldn't get the door open.
Or the estate agent didn't want us to see the contents.
Maybe the Oyster House garage was hiding a pearl
– a beautiful little vintage car dating back to the
1930's. An Austin 7 Pearl Cabriolet, the soft top and
seats now sadly rotted, and bodywork rusted. A home
to generations of spiders.

It wasn't the young estate agent, Beatrice from Bees
Homes, with honey blonde hair. She was pleasant
enough, and didn't buzz around with sales talk.
*And* she was very sweet to me, so I smiled and
made polite comments. But not too positive, so she
wouldn't think she'd made a sale. I couldn't tell
what Ben was thinking. He didn't say much. I think
that spoke volumes.

It was when I was alone. Sitting in the kitchen, on
the wooden stool with a wobbly leg, that I had this
feeling. A feeling of *overwhelming sadness* when I
opened a cupboard, within arms reach of where I
perched. Just an empty cupboard. Bare. Boring. A
lonely space. A grey hole in the kitchen universe.
But my eye was drawn to a poster blue-tacked to
the inside of the cupboard door. It was of a tranquil
beach. A tropical paradise. Clear waters. Golden
sands. Palm trees. Reminding me of the comedy-
drama, *Shirley Valentine*. Shirley had longed to
escape from a mundane life with her boring, gruff
husband. She would find herself talking to the kitchen
wall, and would open a kitchen cupboard, with a
poster on the inside of the door of a beach in Greece.

She had dreamt of travelling abroad since she was young, and finally, in her forties, found the courage to go on holiday to Greece with a friend – but never returned home, because she found herself a job and started to make a new life there, on her own.

The woman who lived in this house had *dreamed*. But never left. I wanted to rest my head in my arms and weep. I must have felt her spirit. I thought for a moment, I *really* would drown under waves of sadness. And my heart sink to the deepest ocean. A single tear trickled down my cheek and splashed onto world-weary-white Formica. And all I could think was – *Is this really happening?*

The Oyster House had been hiding a lonely pearl. She had made her bed. And must lie in it.

\* \* \* \* \* \* \* \*

BEN:      So, what do you think dear?

ME:       I need a drink.

\* \* \* \* \* \* \* \*

The Ocean View café didn't have an ocean view. Well, it may have from an upstairs room, or if you stood on the toilet and peered out of a small window. I didn't care. It was friendly, homely and peaceful (only two other softly spoken couples), and a delicious smell drifted out of the kitchen. *And* it was pleasantly warm. Most welcome after a very chilly walk from the seafront car park, where I saw a ginger cat intently watching a seagull, larger than itself, plodding on the pebbles. I've never seen a cat on a beach before.

We found a table for two in a cosy corner, next to a pine dresser with shelves full of enticing jars. Honey and jams, the colours of autumn. Delicious looking golds, crimsons, reds and blackcurrant, in shiny jars with white mop-cap tops. Everything looking beautifully, wonderfully *clean and shiny,* after the visit to the grubby, neglected house – the cutlery on the red and white check tablecloth, the white, wooden chairs we sat on, the white china cups we drank our tea from, the floor, and the walls, adorned with little colourful paintings for sale by local artists, in white frames.

I sat silently for a while, just sipping raspberry tea and admiring the artworks. The café had run out of peppermint tea, so I decided I would *try to like* the raspberry. Ben drank normal tea. No de-caf or herbal for him. Proper tea.

BEN:      How's the raspberry tea?

ME:        I'm trying to find something I like about it.

BEN:      Like the Oyster House.

ME:        Yes.

BEN:      It's a nice raspberry colour.

ME:        Very-tea-red.

BEN:      Mine's very-tea-brown.

ME:        You're drinking *proper tea* after visiting a *property*.

29

BEN:     Yes dear.

ME:      The artworks in here are inspiring me to paint. If we find a lovely home by he sea, I'll paint seagulls.

BEN:     I admire your creativi-*tea* (pointing to teacup).

ME:      Thanks (smiling tiredly).

BEN:     And *we will* find a lovely home.

ME:      I admire your positivi-*tea*.

## WE SIP IN SILENCE

ME:      Did you know, the man who invented painting by numbers, got the idea from Leonardo da Vinci, who used the technique to help train his students?

BEN:     Extraordinary dear.

ME:      I knew a girl at school. Nice, quiet girl. Claire. We called her Clarinety Claire.

BEN:     She played the clarinet.

ME:      Yes. Anyway, we became friends and one day I visited her at her home. There was a painting by numbers of horses that she had done, framed and hung over the fireplace. Her parents were proud of their only child's achievement. I remember thinking – how lovely! I admired the artwork, and decided I'd like to do a painting by numbers. But I never did (yawning sleepily).

BEN:     Would you like a painting by numbers kit?

ME: I don't know (tired sigh).

BEN: Maybe Santa will get you one for Christmas.

ME: That would be nice, horses would be good (sip, sip, yawn).

BEN: Or a cat.

ME: Yes. A cat (smiling sleepily).

BEN: The chocolate cake here looks good, but I mustn't be tempted.

ME: There was another Claire at school, the boys called her Chocolaty Claire.

BEN: Did she love chocolate?

ME: She had chocolate brown skin – chocolate éclair, you know – the sweets.

BEN: Did she mind?

ME: No, because she was pretty and the boys fancied her. And everyone thought she was very sweet.

WE LAUGH


## Sunday 11th

11.00 a.m. Sitting on the bed.

11.01 a.m. Wearily watching the flags around the building site, advertising the wonderful new housing estate, flapping in the wind. There are no workmen plodding about in their muddy wellies today, so I'm enjoying the peace.

11.02 a.m.  Some of the mounds of earth and rubble have flat tops, bringing to mind dormant volcanos. One of the mounds brings to mind the burial mounds I saw on *Time Team*. The mound nearest our house is as high as — I don't know what.

11.03 a.m.  As high as halfway up our bedroom window. It's a small mountain.

11.05 a.m.  The sky is volcano ash grey.

11.06 a.m.  I feel burnt out.

11.07 a.m.  Flat.

ME:  There are volcanoes, a burial mound and mountains on the building site.

BEN:  That's nice dear.

* * * * * * * *

11.32 a.m.  Lying on the bed.

11.33 a.m.  Diamanda is just being a cat, curled up in the bedroom window, yawning a big-cat-yawn. She is enjoying the peace too (no twitching tail or owl ears). As I watch her, I yawn a big-cat-yawn (no twitching mouth or sad tears). Cats teach you how to yawn *really well*.

11.36 a.m.  I watch a pigeon swoop onto a mountain top.

11.37 a.m.  I sigh a *big sigh*. Exhaustion swooping and landing on my shoulders, like a great big eagle with claws of fatigue. And I'm starting to feel there are not just mountains on the building site, the house is full of them.

ME:  The house is full of mountains and mounds.

BEN:  Is it? (slightly concerned frown).

ME:  Yes. Mountains of washing-up to be done – great walls of china. Mounds of dust. Piles of paperwork. Huge mountain ranges of clothes need washing. You'll have to conquer them for me at the moment. I have no army left. They all died in battle or deserted me.

BEN:  Yes dear.

1.00 p.m.  Sitting on the sofa.

1.01 p.m.  TV Weekly on lap.

1.02 p.m.  I see *Extreme Everest With Ant Middleton* is on tonight. An adrenalin-fuelled account of ex-special forces hero Ant's attempt to climb the highest mountain on earth. The ascent proves a more daunting challenge than anything he's faced in his military career.

1.03 p.m.  Hmm. If he thinks that's daunting, he should be me, climbing thirteen steps up the stairs to the bathroom. On a bad day.

1.05 p.m.  Maybe I'll watch *Harry And Megan: The First Tour.* The Duke and Duchess of Sussex will be on a sixteen day trip across the South Pacific, visiting Australia, Fiji, Tonga and New Zealand. I'll watch just to see any animals they may encounter – hopefully some Koala bears.

1.06 p.m.  There's a romantic Christmas film on at the same time, *Christmas Under Wraps* – a teacher moves to a remote Alaskan location and discovers that the small town is hiding a big secret. Maybe I'll doze to that instead.

1.07 p.m.  Smile to myself as I recall a name a teacher gave a girl at school called Carol – Christmas Carol.

1.08 p.m.  There's another romantic Christmas film on a bit later, *My Christmas Prince* – a woman discovers her European diplomat boyfriend Callum Alexander, is secretly heir to his country's throne. What shall I watch? *Decisions, decisions.*

1.09 p.m.  I'm all decided. Will watch (mostly doze to) Harry and Megan on their adventure abroad. Then *My Christmas Prince* – for a *right* royal romantic afternoon.

1.10 p.m.  Tonight I'll watch *Mega Volcano: Draining the Pacific*. Under the Pacific Ocean lies a vast area known as the Ring of Fire, where seventy-five percent of the world's volcanos lie and ninety percent of earthquakes occur. The documentary, based on the latest ocean floor maps, uses visual effects to 'drain' the ocean and reveal the geological forces behind some of the Earth's most destructive natural disasters. Ooh, that sounds a *very scary* place. I wouldn't want to sail my little boat across the Ring of Fire. If I had a little boat.

1.20 p.m.    Standing in the Kitchen, stirring hot carrot and lentil soup in a saucepan. Singing quietly to myself – the chorus of a song from the sixties about a ring of fire, although I don't think Johnny Cash was singing about a ring of volcanos under the Pacific Ocean.

> *I fell into a burning ring of fire,*
> *I went down, down, down, and the flames went higher*
> *And it burn, burns, burns*
> *The ring of fire, the ring of fire.*

BEN:    I'm off into town now.

ME:    Are you getting a *round-tuit?*

BEN:    If I can find one. I'll be popping into Sainsbury's, want anything?

ME:    Mm, something fit for a chocolate loving princess.

BEN:    Chocolate tiara?

ME:    I'm too hot headed, it would melt. I'm like a little volcano, wanting to erupt with bedroom – I mean boredom.

BEN:    I'll surprise you with a little something dear.

## Monday 12th

9.00 a.m.    It *would* be today wouldn't it. *Today of all days!* That I accidentally knocked over a mug. A whole mug. Not the last few slurps. *Or* quarter of a mug. *Or* half a mug. NO. It had to be a whole ruddy mug of coffee, tipped into my underwear drawer. On a day when I'm feeling delayed fatigue after Saturday's exertions. And one *really does* not want brown stains on one's white delicates. Or the pretty pastel lacy ones. And of course, there *would be,* at the bottom of the drawer, a catalogue selling Christmassy under-wear, completely drenched, and stuck to soggy, moggy and froggy socks... *Is this really happening?*

9.30 a.m.    Lying on bed. Exhausted. Listening to the rumbling sound of the washing machine. And the caterpillar tracks on the building site. Praying something nice will happen.

10.11 a.m.    KNOCK! KNOCK! KNOCK!

ME:    *Hurrah!* The draught-proof curtains have arrived. My prayers have been answered.

BEN:    Your prayers?

ME:    I wanted something nice to happen. Anything. The arrival of curtains will do. And we'll have a cosier kitchen, now you've bought another *round-tuit.*

BEN:    And I will get around to putting them up. Do you like the colour?

ME:    Love it. *Love it!* Delicious. Belgian-dark-chocolate brown.

BEN:    Thought you'd approve. Will I come home one day and find you chewing the curtains?

ME:    Maybe. On a bad day! Or when you forget to tell me you'll be home *really* late and I start to worry as the hours drag by....... But I must admit, I want to lick them now, they're shiny and satin-smooth, like those Galaxy chocolate buttons, with a crispy coating.

BEN: You must have one of the treats I gave you yesterday.

ME: Mm, I will. Those Belgian chocolate seahorses are *sea-sational!*

11.07 a.m. *KNOCK! KNOCK! KNOCK!* – on next door's front door.

11.09 a.m. Sounds like people are viewing the house to rent. *I'm so relieved* the previous tenants have moved out. They were another reason we want to move, they were *so noisy and stressful.* And for some reason, Asian people screaming and shouting all the time, sounds worse than the British. Maybe it's just that I'm a nosey neighbour, and frustrated because I don't know what they are fighting about.

ME: I hope the new neighbours will be quieter than the last ones.

BEN: We'll have to wait and see.

ME: Oh God (big sigh), there have been *so many* awful people renting next door since dear old Maurice and Jean moved to a home without stairs, to make their life easier. To begin their journey. Tread their first step on the stairway to heaven. It's been *eight very long* years.

Maurice is in heaven now, I know he will be, he was such a nice, gentle man. I still send a Christmas card to Jean, and she sent us a lovely one with a robin on last year, did I show it to you?

BEN:    I can't remember (weary look).

ME:    Do you remember that young couple, she was an air hostess, a flighty sort, with fly-away blonde hair. Worked odd hours. He seemed rather timid. And there would be lots of shouting in the early hours. Although not as bad as the couple the other side who used to throw things, and we could hear all the crashing sounds. *And* although it was disturbing, *at least* I could be nosey and hear what they were fighting about – usually jealousy or money. And then one day the air hostess wasn't there anymore, and the man was laying a patio. He did a nice job, I could see it if I stood on the side of the bath and peered out of the top of the bathroom window. The slabs were different colours, very creative I thought. Sort of blonde yellow and angry-girl-pink.

BEN:    I remember (smiling).

ME:    Then there was that *weirdo*. Ugh. I shudder at the memory. I never *actually saw* him, but he was a constant creepy presence for almost a year. Always standing at his back door, only a few feet away from me when I was in the kitchen. Maybe I could have seen him if I'd peered through one of the little round holes in the fence, but imagine if an evil eye stared back at me – *I shudder at the thought.*

BEN:    How did you know he was there?

ME:    His horrible cigarette smoke would waft into our kitchen in the summer, when our back door was open. And the stench seeped in through the edges of the door when it was closed. I *just felt* he wasn't a nice person. I'd often hear him sniff or make an evil growly sort of cough. And sometimes I could *feel* him *listening,* in an evil I-hate-women way, to me talking to you or one of our cats, or singing to myself. And he didn't like it when I laughed.

BEN: When you did one of your *very witchy* cackles.

ME: Yes. I would suddenly stop, mid-cackle, and my witchy sense would tell me he was listening in a disapproving way, followed by a strong whiff of foul smelling fag........ *foul smelling fag blown at the hag, when the neighbour takes a drag.*

BEN: Do you feel a poem coming on?

ME: No. Not today.

BEN: The landlady told me he never paid his rent.

ME: I knew he was a *bad-un.*

BEN: There was the couple with the dog that barked a lot, and the couple with little girl who cried all the time, and they were always shouting at each other.

ME: *And* always making-up, because I heard her say on her mobile phone to a friend that *they* were at-it-like-rabbits. Then the next thing we knew, there was a baby boy with a *very* powerful pair of lungs, that I'm sure the whole street could hear.

BEN: Then endless *fighting, screaming, crying.*

ME: I was *SO* relieved when they moved away. I think after that there was a foreign couple. They were OK. I *loved* the smell of their oily, spicy food drifting out of their kitchen window. Then after that another foreign couple. Not so nice. Had to call the police when you were away.

BEN: Don't remind me.

\* \* \* \* \* \* \* \*

12.20 p.m. I'm reading an article in Celebrity Weekly entitled, *We rented a digger and the kids loved it.*

ME: Peter Andre and his wife Emily have rented a digger, because they're going to plant some trees and hedges in their front garden. It's a miniature version of the ones on the building site, look at the photo, it looks fun!

BEN: Now you want me to rent a miniature digger, so you can join in with the workmen on the building site, for a bit of fun.

ME: Well, if you can't beat 'em!

BEN: What are you like.

ME: I *do wish* lots of trees were going to be planted, instead of houses. An old friend of mine said the car park was once an orchard.

BEN: So that's why we're Orchard Street.

ME: Yes, but I'm going to re-name it now.

BEN:      Let me guess. Orrible Street? Noisy Street?

ME:       Wish-it-was-an-orchard Street.

BEN:      I quite agree dear.


## Tuesday 13th

8.25 a.m.    I'm in the kitchen, perched on a stool, sleepily watching golden-yellow leaves flying wildly across the lavender-blue sky. I sip hot minty tea as the squirrels stuff their little grey, whiskery faces with peanuts on the bird table, then scamper off to bury them, here and there on the lawn. When they are busy *dig, dig, digging* in the grass, the tiny birds appear on the table for a tasty nibble.

8.27 a.m.    I enjoy a toasty nibble.

9.20 a.m.    I'm in the bedroom, perched on the bed, sleepily watching dark green flags around the building site, fluttering in the breeze. They bring to mind the spooky wraiths in the Harry Potter films.

9.21 a.m.    Oh God!

9.22 a.m.    It looks like there's a skull sticking out of a pile of rubble on the building site. And close by there's two finger bones sticking out.

9.24 a.m.    Phew! It's OK. Panic over – now that I'm wearing my distance glasses, I see the finger bones are tree roots, and the skull is a lump of concrete. I've been watching too much archaeology. Too much digging up of skeletons on Tony's *Time Team*.

10.03 a.m.    I'm in the bathroom, perched on the side of the bath, like a saggy bag of archaeologist's ancient bits of bone and pottery. I'm deep in thought – deep as one of Tony's *Time Team* trenches.

10.05 a.m.    I'm slumped. Like an archaeologist at the end of a long, tiring dig, in the middle of nowhere, in the middle of winter, with no interesting finds. Not one single piece of pottery, bone or mosaic piece.

10.10 a.m.    Staring in bathroom mirror. I'm pale as ashes found in a pottery pot on *Time Team*.

10.11 a.m.    I don't feel *grate*.

10.30 a.m.    Maybe I'll watch another romantic Christmas film, *A Cinderella Christmas* on Channel 5. Or the drama, *Ashes to Ashes* on Drama Channel. Or a Sci-fi film, *The Day the Earth Caught Fire* on Sony Movie Channel. Or a thriller, *Inferno* (sequel to *Angels and Demons)* on BBC 1.

10.32 a.m.    I'm *far too* tired to be thrilled, or enjoy *too much* drama or romance. Will watch my usual viewing, followed by a nice sleepy house-buying programme, *Coast Vs Country*.

* * * * * * * *

3.00 p.m.    After watching a repeat of last night's *Coronation Street* – Claudia surprised Audrey at the Stylist's Awards by saying unkind things. Audrey threw a bouquet of flowers in Claudia's face, and Claudia fell over backwards in her chair (lots of drama, but not too much drama for a tired person). And *Time Team* – Tony and his team excavated a Neolithic

42

henge in Durrington, near Stonehenge. They found some interesting finds, including deer antlers used for construction. And it was exciting when they found a connection between the two sites – the river Avon (but not too exciting for a tired person). I then curled up with Diamanda and dozed to *Coast Vs Country*.

3.02 p.m.   A couple – a teacher and an import operator (whatever that is), are searching for a property in Suffolk. The teacher wants to live by the coast, and her husband wants to live in the country. The house in the country is beautiful, with lots of character, in a peaceful village with a cosy country pub. The property by the coast is very handsome, with windswept sandy beaches – named The Amber Coast because of the fossils. Let's see who gets their wish.

3.03 p.m.   If they choose the coast, that means Ben and I will find a nice home by the sea. Fingers crossed.

3.04 p.m.   Toes crossed.

3.05 p.m.   Eyes crossed.

3.06 p.m.   Broomsticks crossed.

3.25 p.m.   They are keeping us in suspense. The teacher is getting a bit cross.

3.30 p.m.   I'm on the edge of the sofa. Legs crossed. Biting a finger nail.

3.40 p.m.   I need to visit the bathroom. They must not decide without me. I will hang on. I *can't miss* the end.

3.45 p.m.   It's no good. I need to go *now*.

3.46 p.m.   I'll be as quick as I can.

3.47 p.m.   While I'm sitting on the loo the house shakes, so the loo is shaking under me. Most disconcerting. I think to myself, it must be like this on a ship, or if you need *to go* on a train, and I forget I'm in a hurry to get back to the TV.

3.55 p.m.   What? The programme can't be over!

3.56 p.m.   *NO! NO! NO!*

3.57 p.m.   Life can be so cruel.

3.58 p.m.   I need a *whole* chocolate cake.

3.59 p.m.   I wonder if the couple came to a decision. Or they are now divorced. The teacher was looking *very cross* at times, like she was dealing with a class full of delinquents, and wasn't sure how to handle them. And the import man thought *his view* was the most important.

4.00 p.m.   I don't think they will ever find their dream home. Maybe we'll never find our dream home by the sea.

4.01 p.m.   I need a whole chocolate cake, smothered in chocolate ice cream, drizzled with chocolate sauce and single cream, sprinkled with chocolate flakes and hazelnuts.

4.02 p.m.   Wholemeal toast smothered with cottage cheese, sprinkled with chopped chives and ground black pepper will do. A much healthier alternative.

4.07 p.m.   Munching cheese on toast, watching *A Place In The Sun* – Homes with beautiful blue-flag beaches in

Crete, enjoyed by happy families in the sun. A thousand miles away. A thousand times better than a view of a green-flag-surrounded building site, endured by angry workmen, in the cold.

4.20 p.m.     Diamanda is snoozing and purring on TV Weekly, peaceful as palm trees in a tropical breeze. A puss in paradise.

4.21 p.m.     I want to know what's on TV tonight, but I don't want to disturb her.

4.23 p.m.     *Crash! Crash! Crash!* Clitter, clatter, clitter, clatter, of caterpillar tracks. The house shakes violently. So the coffee table shakes too. And Diamanda, curled up on TV Weekly (on the coffee table), is shaken out of her sweet dream world.

4.24 p.m.     Diamanda decides my lap will be a safer place.

4.25 p.m.     As she purrs, I peruse TV Weekly.

4.26 p.m.     Ooh, I see there's a must-watch on Channel 4 tonight – *The Crossrail Discovery: London's Lost Graveyard*. The discovery of a lost 17th Century burial site, exposed in a rail line dig.

\* \* \* \* \* \* \* \* \*

5.00 p.m.

ME:          I'd loved to have visited the Tunnel exhibition at the Docklands Museum last year.

BEN:         Toenail exhibition?

ME: Tunnel (grinning). Remember the Crossrail discovery?

BEN: Oh yeah, all the skeletons.

ME: And lots of artefacts were found dating back eight thousand years – hundreds of interesting finds. Tony and his team of archaeologists on *Time Team* would have been very excited to have dug up things like Roman horseshoes, Medieval bone ice skates, Victorian chamber pots, a leather shoe dating back to the fifteenth or sixteenth Century, and woolly mammoth bones. I'd liked to have seen them.

BEN: Never mind dear, maybe they'll discover something interesting on the building site. The grave of King Richard the third was discovered under a car park a few years ago, when an archaeologist was excavating the ruins of a monastery in Leicester.

ME: I don't suppose his spirit was happy when dirty great, noisy, *horseless chariots* parked over his head in the car park. Then people climbed out of the chariots, slamming doors – *bang!... bang!... bang!* And a bit later, returned with Sainsbury's carrier bags, and made *more* noise – the rumbling of engines making his poor old bones shake.

BEN: Like our bones when work starts in our once-was-a-car park.

ME: Yes (half smiling and nodding). Anyway, I'll look out for a pointy crown sticking out of the rubble.

## Wednesday 14th

9.20 a.m.

ME: My stars say I should focus on my hopes and wishes, and try picturing myself where I'd like to be in five or ten years time. Cosmic Colin says this will act as an anchor by which to navigate future decisions.

BEN: I imagine you don't see yourself dropping anchor near the Oyster Houses in Pevensey Bay.

ME: No, but the Ocean View Café was nice. Maybe I'd drop anchor for a cuppa and slice of cake.

BEN: What do my stars say?

ME: Scorpio – this week you need to focus on household chores. This will be beneficial for your health because the extra exercise will do you good. Help you lose more weight. *Especially* if you hoover the stairs, clean the bathroom basin, toilet and cooker, empty the food bin, take out the recycling, de-frost the fridge and de-flea Diamanda.

BEN: That's clever of Colin to know we've got a cat *dear*.

\* \* \* \* \* \* \* \*

10.05 a.m. Leafing through today's TV viewing (like a lady of leisure, while Ben scrubs the cooker), I see *Homes By The Sea* is on at 2 p.m. The presenter will be in a place I like on the South Coast, not that far from Pevensey – appeals to me because it's bohemian and a little surreal. We visited there after we'd viewed a few bungalows (from the outside) at nearby St Mary's

Bay and Lydd.

11.03 p.m.    Ben is collapsed on sofa after cleaning the bathroom basin and toilet, taking out the recycling rubbish and food bin, de-fleaing Diamanda *and* refreshing her litter tray. The basin and toilet weren't *that* grubby. And there were only two little bags of recycling. And not *too* many poohs in the litter tray. *And* Diamanda is fairly good at coping with a de-flea. But I make him a coffee and a snack because men need a reward after doing lots of little jobs. Especially ones they don't want to do – which makes them emotionally stressed. Well, that's in my experience anyway.

1.14 p.m.    I exclaim enthusiastically, and in a *most heartfelt* manner, how lovely the staircase looks, now it's clean – as I slump, sitting on the seventh step up, head resting on the tired, threadbare coffee brown carpet, hoping *with all my heart* for some energy to climb the next six steps. Because men need praise and encouragement after toiling in a house doing *women's* work.

2.15 p.m.    I'm watching *Homes By The Sea*.

ME:    Recognise this place? (pointing to TV screen).

BEN:    No.

ME:    Dungeness. We went there when we were lookin' at houses nearby in Lydd. Remember?

BEN:    Oh. Yeah.

ME:    I like Dungeness, it has such a surreal feel. Remote.

Other worldly. Some of the homes are renovated railway carriages from the nineteen thirties. I like the way the homes are dotted about, with no order, like sandcastles on a beach, different sizes and shapes. Each one unique.

BEN: Would you like to live there?

ME: The place did appeal to me. Attracts eccentric arty types –

BEN: Like you.

ME: Yes (nodding), I feel *drawn* to the place, but (frowning a little) –

BEN: The grim view of Dungeness Power Station didn't inspire you.

ME: Or you! Gave me the creeps. A feeling of impending doom. Probably because I recall that disaster back in the eighties, when a nuclear power station safety test went wrong in the Ukraine, and radioactive smoke and dust was unleashed across Europe.

BEN: Chernobyl.

ME: Yes. Dreadful.

BEN: Yeah.

ME: And Dungeness feels like a place artists go to die (smiling gravely). Probably because I remember, in the eighties again, reading about an artist living there who was dying of aids. He created little metal sculptures in his garden. It made me feel so sad. I wonder

49

if they still exist.

BEN:       Rusting in peace.

ME:        Yes. Oh, and would you believe, there's an architect who lives there now, who built his home, the whole interior, inspired by the power station. He has a window that *actually frames* the view of the station. Apparently it looks beautiful at sunset!

BEN:       Shocking dear.... Bill used to go there.

ME:        The power station? Your artist mate Bill?

BEN:       Yeah.

ME:        He wasn't inspired to paint it, was he?

BEN:       No (laughing), when he had his driving job, delivering nuts and bolts. He said when he delivered to other places there were numerous check points, and you needed a pass. But at the power station there was just a little old man in a shed who said, 'Alright Bill!'

* * * * * * * *

3.00 p.m.

BEN:       Minty tea?

ME:        Mm, please.

3.06 p.m.

BEN:       Here you are dear.

50

ME: Ah, just my cup of tea.

BEN: Unlike Dungeness.

ME: And the raspberry tea at Pevensey Bay.

BEN: We did see some *proper teas* on the south coast we liked though.

ME: Yes, ones you and Bill hadn't viewed from the out-side. I wasn't feeling too bad at the time, so thought I'd have a bit of fun, on an afternoon out with you, trying to find them. The photos looked good on the internet. Remember Lydd?

BEN: Refresh my memory (sipping his refreshment).

ME: We had a bit of trouble finding the property, and when I eventually spotted it, it looked OK. *But* some of the neighbouring bungalows looked dilapidated, with junk in the front gardens and dirty looking curtains. A bit of a rough area, with youths kicking footballs in the road, and we almost got a ball in our windscreen.

BEN: *Don't-come-and-live-in-our-road-with-your-posh-French-car* (laughing).

ME: I didn't need to *see* the neighbours.

BEN: I remember the neighbour we *did see.*

ME: Oh, yes. The attached property in St Mary's Bay. And what a beautiful bay. I can't believe we have so many lovely bays on the south coast that I've never visited!

BEN: Yeah.

ME: The St Mary's Bay semi-detached bungalow was another one that was a bit difficult to locate, because it was on a corner with a hedge all around it. So I got quite excited, when I finally spotted it in a quiet, well maintained area. Looked really peaceful. Birdies were twittering happily in the trees. A well fed tabby cat plodded nonchalantly by. And we got out of the car to cross the little green to have a closer look.

BEN: You liked it until the neighbour emerged from the attached property.

ME: Oh yes. The man with the air of aggression, Alsation dog, and *Dungenession* grimness.

BEN: You and your made-up words!

ME: But it's a good description, you have to agree.

BEN: I do dear.

ME: And he had a *don't-you-move-next-door-to-me* look on his ex-con-like face.

BEN: Maybe he is an ex-con.

ME: His expression and body language suggested he could easily creep in our back door, after nipping through the broken fence, and murder me while you are out. Or poison our cat, because he hates cats. Or set his huge Alsation on our cat, or on me, to bite my legs off, or hold a gun to my head – just because I politely requested he turn the volume of his *Guns and Roses* rock music down at two o'clock in the

morning, and picked a shell pink rose from a neglected rose bush, that was leaning over his fence
into our garden. I couldn't resist, the scent was so
delightful. A scent he hated (and loathed seeing me
swoon at the fragrance) because it reminded him of
his mother's perfume, whom he had murdered and
buried next to the rose bush, that she had planted
and tended with care and affection. An affection she
had never been able to show him, because he was
too much like his evil father, who died in prison
serving a life sentence for killing three young women,
who reminded him of his mother.

BEN:      You and your imagination!

ME:      Well, you just don't know. You won't read *that sort
of thing* on a website selling properties. Nor would
you read some of the other things we discovered.

BEN:      Remind me.

ME:      There was a detached bungalow in the same area
that looked good on the internet photos, with a big,
well maintained front lawn. But it turned out to be
on the corner of a busy crossroads, with a busier
roundabout nearby.

BEN:      Oh yeah. And there was some sort of youth club,
with a graffiti covered basketball area, next to the
front lawn.

ME:      And I imagined it getting noisy, with basket balls
flying over the fence into our garden, and young men
always knocking on the door asking to retrieve their
ball. Or just jumping over our hedge to retrieve a
ball, and maybe flattening the daffodils with their

Doc Martin boots.

BEN: Maybe the club is full of juvenile delinquents, who will threaten you if you tell them off for flattening your flowers. Or murder you when I'm out, because they are like their ex-con fathers. And two of them are the sons of the aggressive ex-con looking neighbour we saw (smiling).

ME: Well you just *don't know*, do you.

BEN: No dear, they won't tell you *that sort of thing* on a property website.

## Thursday 15th

10.58 a.m. On the building site, rubble is scooped up and tipped into a skip.

10.59 a.m. In my kitchen I scoop de-caf coffee granules out of a jar and tip into the cafetière.

11.00 a.m. The washing machine rumbles to the end of its cycle.

11.01 a.m. The rumbling on the building site is making the house shake so much, I feel like I'm sitting on a washing machine, during the final spin.

11.02 a.m. A digger plunges into dark grey ground, as I press down the plunger in my cafetière – breathing in the aroma of ground coffee beans.

11.03 a.m. I pour coffee into a mug.

11.04 a.m.   Broken up concrete is poured into a skip.

11.05 a.m.   The house trembles. The surface of my coffee quivers.

12.01 p.m.   A workman climbs out of a deep trench for his lunch break.

12.05 p.m.   Archaeologists are climbing into trenches on *Time Team*. They've discovered Roman pottery and skeletons next to a church.

12.15 p.m.   Archaeologist Faye, complains to Tony from the bottom of her heart (I mean trench), that her hole has nothing in it. After *all* the effort she's put in, with *all* her heart.

Never mind Faye, there are worse things in life.

12.30 p.m.   Caterpillar tracks have stopped rumbling on the building site, but my tummy rumbles on, in need of a lunchtime snack. Like the end of an archaeolgical dig, it's a hole that needs filling.

12.31 p.m.   Rubble has been taken from a huge triangular mound and spread evenly over earth.

12.32 p.m.   I evenly spread a small triangle of Dairy Lee cheese onto wholemeal toast. Then top with sliced tomato, sprinkled with pepper.

1.03 p.m.   The digging continues, now the workmen have returned from their lunch break. I watch *Loose Women* after my lunchtime snack. This week is Retro Week – lots of amusing clips taken from 1970's and 1980's sitcoms.

1.05 p.m.    I enjoy a much needed laugh.

1.10 p.m.    Workmen laugh when a colleague trips over a rock and falls into a puddle. Splash!

1.15 p.m.    The women on the *Loose Women* panel laugh with embarrassment when clips of them are shown from the 1980's – lots of big hair, big jewellery and shoulder pads.

1.17 p.m.    A JCB whines and snorts.

1.18 p.m.    On *Loose Women,* Janet Street-Porter whines and snorts. I like her. She always makes me giggle.

2.15 p.m.    Rocks are being broken up.

2.16 p.m.    In a repeat of *Coronation Street*, Abi feels broken. Her life is falling apart because of Tracey.

2.20 p.m.    A digger digs deep to clear away the demolished showroom.

2.21 p.m.    In *Coronation Street*, Nick digs deep into his pocket to pay Carla to keep quiet, Leanne still has no idea he is married.

2.22 p.m.    What *on earth* is Nick thinking.

2.23 p.m.    Rocks continue to be broken up.

3.01 p.m.    I read in TV Weekly that Leanne and Nick may be breaking-up in tomorrow's episode. Leanne is going to find out he is married, *I just know it!*

3.30 p.m.    Our house shakes violently as metal jaws crash into the ground.

3.31 p.m.     In *Most Haunted,* Yvette and her team are sitting around a table doing a seance in a most haunted museum, and the table is starting to shake as a violent spirit begins to communicate with them.

3.32 p.m.     Our house shakes again, and for a moment I shudder at the thought of a violent spirit making this happen.

3.34 p.m.     The spirit whispers nastily in Yvette's ear, 'Get lost', and things are being thrown across the room. Yvette's going to start screaming. *I just know it!*

3.43 p.m.     Ben bursts in through the front door, stamping his wet boots on the doormat, and I let out a little scream of fear.

BEN:     You're jumpy!

ME:     I'm watching *Most Haunted.*

BEN:     Ah, should've guessed.

ME:     Sounds like it's *really* chucking it down out there.

BEN:     Yep (unzipping his drenched jacket).

ME:     It'll get even muddier on the building site. I saw a workman fall on his face in a muddy puddle today.

BEN:     And you couldn't help laughing.

ME:     Yes, especially when a lot of bad words came out of his mouth...... Do you know what a mudlark is?

BEN:        A man larking about in the mud?

ME:         No.

BEN:        A type of wading bird?

ME:         A person who plods about scavenging for objects of interest or value on a riverbed – I heard a woman on the radio last night talking about her hobby. She goes out at night with a torch at low tide, on the bed of the Thames river, finds lots of things,  then brings them home to dry out!

BEN:        I expect you're going to tell me all the *arty facts*.

ME:         They were quite interesting. She finds Roman coins, jewellery, hairpins and mosaic pieces. She found a very rare sword scabbard once. There's lots of pottery, clay pipes, and shoes dating back to the sixteenth and seventeenth century in her collection too – all sorts.

BEN:        Were they liquorice?


## Friday 16th

5.00 p.m.

ME:         *Oh God! Oh God!* There's a hand sticking out of a pile of rubble on the building site. A body has been buried! They may have been *buried alive!*

BEN:        Are you sure dear? (yawning).

ME:         *YES!* Look for yourself – there! (pointing to a pile of rubble, nearest our bedroom window).

BEN:      Yeah, I see it.

ME:       There was a disagreement on the building site today,
          it got quite heated at one point. *VERY HEATED!* Lots
          of arm waving, finger pointing, stomping around,
          and swearing. Maybe a workman has *murdered* one
          of his colleagues, and is planning to throw the body
          into a trench and pour concrete over the top. And
          the ghost will wander across our street and haunt
          our house for eternity!

BEN:      You've been watching too much *Columbo* and *Most
          Haunted*. Put your distance glasses on dear.

ME:       Ah. Silly me. It's a white rubber glove.

BEN:      Maybe you need a bit of drama in your life. There's
          a double bill of *Agatha Christie's Poirot* on tonight.

ME:       Oh, goody.

                        * * * * * * * * *

5.20 p.m.   Perusing TV Weekly, I find the Agatha Christie dou-
            ble bill. *The King of Clubs*: An actress witnesses
            the murder of a shady producer, only to become the
            prime suspect. And *The Dream*: A well known eccen-
            tric contacts the Belgian sleuth when he's haunted
            by suicidal nightmares – Lots of lovely drama.

5.22 p.m.   I notice, *Skeletons Of The Mary Rose: The New
            Evidence,* is on at 9 p.m. Scientists use isotope and
            DNA technology to analyse the human remains found
            on Henry VIII's iconic war ship which sank in 1545

– and the results challenge ideas that Tudor England was a white homogeneous monoculture. They also trace descendants of two of the crew members whose names are known – Sounds interesting.

5.30 p.m.

ME: Kirstie Allsopp said a funny house-moving-word on *Location, Location, Location* today. I expect she made it up herself, she's got a great sense of humour.

BEN: Do tell me, I'm eager to know.

ME: She said she wanted a young couple, Anna and Mike, to find a wish-list-tick-tastick house!

BEN: No doubt you'll be using that word now.

ME: I'll probably add a bit. Wish-list-tick-tastic-seasidey-sensation.

BEN: Doesn't surprise me dear.

7.10 p.m.

ME: The chocolate brown curtains over the back door, make the kitchen look *and* feel warm and cosy. When the house looks lovely we won't want to leave!

BEN: Yeah. Come and look in the cellar.

ME: Must I? I'm SO tired.

BEN: You'll be surprised.

ME: OK.... Successful spray job?

BEN:     Yep. The white cistern is now avocado green.

＊ ＊ ＊ ＊ ＊ ＊ ＊ ＊

ME:     Oh yes! Another successful *round-tuit*. The spray paint has worked really well. It'll look good when you've installed it in the bathroom.

BEN:     It's a darker green than the bath and sink.

ME:     That doesn't matter, it's such a beautiful green. You've done a good job. I never thought I could love a toilet cistern!

BEN:     Thanks. Life is full of little surprises isn't it.

ME:     It certainly, *cisternly* is! That new toilet brush you got – with the best review online, out of the best ten toilet brushes this year, *really is* the best! Cleaning the loo is going to be such a pleasure (feigned, sleepy smile).

BEN:     And it'll be so much more of a pleasure when the next *round-tuit* arrives tomorrow.

ME:     Another *round-tuit*?! (smiling yawn).

BEN:     Yep. It's more of an *oval-shaped-tuit* – toilet seat shaped. Antique pine, with an easy wipe polyurethane, smooth surface, and solid zinc hinges. Five star reviews.

ME:     What did the reviews say?

BEN:     Warm to the bum.... Does a good job!..... And you're gonna love the pink rubber gloves I ordered, for tiny hands. I got a pack of three.

ME:       Lucky me.

BEN:     Yes, they're called Comfies – flock lined, with a rolled cuff, and patterned for grip. They get great reviews too!

ME:       What more could a girl want. Doing the washing-up will be a dream (big yawn).

BEN:     Yeah! (tripping over a can of paint, then bumping into a ladder and knocking it over, so it crashes onto jars of nails and screws, sending the contents flying everywhere). F***.

ME:       Your stars say you'll be faced with obstacles in a new project.

BEN:     Thank you for that information dear.

* * * * * * * *

*Well, we can't stand around here doing nothing, people will think we're workmen.*

Spike Milligan

# December

**Wednesday 5th**

11.46 a.m.    It's a gloomy, drizzly day. But a day I've been looking forward to. We climb into the car. Seat belts on. Ben starts the engine. Checks his mirrors. Then begins to manoeuvre the car out of our parking space, cursing people who park too close.

11.47 a.m.    I feel like we're going on holiday, because it's often a gloomy, drizzly day (and a day I've been looking forward to) when we're off on a holiday.

But we're not going on holiday.

11.48 a.m.    At the end of our street Ben waits for four cars to pass by, before turning the corner and heading for London. As we wait, I spot a notice on the building site fence, with a drawing of the new-estate-to-be.

ME:    Have you seen the seating plan?..... Erm no, I mean floor plan..... I mean –

BEN:    Architect's drawing of the new housing development?

ME:    Yes.

BEN:    I'm afraid so.

ME:    Oh my God! I didn't realise –

BEN:    I know.

ME:    And you didn't want to tell me.

BEN: Yeah.

ME: *Is this really happening?*

BEN: Yes dear.

ME: Oh God... must keep calm...... deep breath....... deep breath...... think of something else.... think.... think. Did you know the Hollywood sign was originally erected in nineteen twenty-three to advertise a housing development?

BEN: No.

ME: It used to read Hollywoodland. That explains the boring lettering, don't you think! As glamorous as a launderette.

BEN: Why a launderette?

ME: I've seen the same lettering over an old launderette, looking very dull – washed out blue on boiled-tea towel white. Next to a Chinese takeaway with bright red and yellow, fancy lettering.

BEN: I fancy a Chinese tonight.

ME: Me too, a treat after our long day. Did you know, the first home delivery service for food, supplied cold noodles in Korea in seventeen sixty-eight?

BEN: You are a mine of wonderful information.

ME: In nineteen forty-nine the Hollywoodland sign was shortened to Hollywood to describe the whole district.

BEN: Very interesting dear.

* * * * * * * *

ME: Flats? A row of *ruddy* flats? Three *ruddy* storeys high? Towering over our little home? I don't believe it!...... *No! No! No!*

BEN: Yep.

ME: Facing our little street – so close, you could hang a washing line between our bedroom window and a window opposite. Will there be a creepy person, dead opposite, watching me? Like the *dead creepy* tenant who stood at his back door listening to me talk in our kitchen? Or maybe the flat owner will think I'm a creepy person watching them, I'm so used to peering out of the window many times a day. And I don't want to change the new lacy curtains that have a gap, so me and Diamanda can watch the world go by.

BEN: Neither do I.

ME: I forgot there would be flats as well as houses, when we were told *ages* ago. They should build them at the far end of the car park, it's just a row of shops, the other side of the road. But I suppose it will be harder to sell flats next to a busy main road, so why not take away the light and a view from our little Victorian terraced houses – all the old people are dying one by one anyway. Why should these architect people care about us over fifties, soon to be in our sixties.

BEN: Yeah.

ME:        Do you know what I have a mind to do?

BEN:      Can't imagine.

ME:        I'll tell you what I have a mind to do!........... Ooh, I suddenly feel very tired. Tell you in a minute (lying down in the back of the car).

BEN:      I'm sure you will dear.

* * * * * * * *

ME:        What I have a mind to do *is* – well, it involves you too.

BEN:      That's nice.

ME:        You'll like it.

BEN:      I'm sure I will dear.

ME:        I want to hand write a letter, with photographs, to our borough council, asking them to forward it to the house planning department. Then I'd like you to e-mail it to them.

BEN:      Photos?

ME:        Yes. I have taken many pics of the view out of our bedroom window. The lovely sunrises I've sat and watched many mornings. And when the car park is empty and covered in a blanket of snow, I've photographed the children building snowmen or having snowball fights – and after the children have gone home, snowmen standing silently, and wonderfully eerie in the winter moonlight..... Colourful, majestic hot air balloons taking flight from the hills around our valley.... Dramatic cloud formations. Rainbows.

BEN:   Fork lightning, as storms travel over our valley.

ME:    I can never manage to capture that on camera, like the fireworks on bonfire night. And the geese flying south for the winter. I'll just have the memories. Anyway, I'd like to write a letter explaining about my illness, and to thank them for taking my view away. Thank them VERY MUCH. Then at the end I'll include a pic of what my view is, when the flats are built.

BEN:   Good idea.

* * * * * * * *

ME:    Guess what?

BEN:   Cold potatoes aren't hot.

ME:    I'm going to stop thinking about it all now, and enjoy my time at the clinic today. Feel chilled. Not so hot headed.

BEN:   Like a hot potato.

ME:    Yes. I'll be a cold potato salad head.

BEN:   And stop letting sad thoughts turn your brain to mash.

ME:    I will, they'll only hinder my bio-energy healing with Seka.

1.10 p.m.   I'm clearing my mind as I watch the clouds, so high in the sky. Far, far away – my grey-cloud thoughts drifting out of the car window, up to meet them. Later the clouds will have drifted far, far away – taking my thoughts with them.

1.12 p.m.     My mind is a clear blue sky.

1.13 p.m.     I sleepily watch a plane making a white trail across the blue, and imagine it is flying to somewhere lovely and warm.

ME:     Leonardo da Vinci said, once you have tasted flight, you will forever walk the earth with your head in the clouds.

BEN:     That's nice dear.

1.15 p.m.     As we approach London's North Circular, the sun begins to appear from behind the clouds.

ME:     Every cloud has a silver lining.

BEN:     Always look on the bright side of life (whistling the tune to *Monty Python's* song about the bright side of life).

ME:     It's always the darkest before the dawn.

* * * * * * * *

2.03 p.m.     **SHOCK! HORROR!** *It's gone completely black! I can't see a thing! I'm trapped! Where's the door? Need to find the handle!.... Can't find the handle! Where is the handle?!... Where is it?!... I'm shaking. Must calm down. Must calm down.... Deep breaths. Must not panic. Must not panic. Must... Not.. Panic.*

2.04 p.m.    ***PANIC! PANIC!*** *I can't breathe!* This tiny toilet cubicle is *SO claustrophobic*. I want to beat my hands on the door and shout – '**HELP!**' But think it would be pointless, there's an outer room with the wash-hand basin, then a corridor with all the doors shut. No-one will hear me. And there's no-one in the waiting area nearby. Ben is searching for a parking space. He could be ages, we *are in London!* And I'll feel silly anyway......... *This blackness so **suffocating**..... Where is the handle?....* Ah. Got it. Didn't expect it to be so low down. It feels stiff. Am I sliding it the wrong way?......... **Phew!** At last, I'm out. But outer room is pitch black too. God, I hate these automatic lights. It's so long since I've been to the clinic, I forgot about them. Vaguely recall, last time I switched the light on when I entered the ladies' room here....... Where is the light switch? Where is the light switch? Is it on the inside of the room? Can't.... find..... light.... switch. Must retrieve handbag. **Where's** my handbag?... Where is it?.... *Where is it?....* Must be next to the toilet. Somehow hold toilet door open and at same time feel around toilet for handbag. Have touched something soft and damp on the floor..... *Ugh..... Horrible!*

2.05 p.m.    Got handbag! Right. Must find door of outer room. MUST find way out of here. Can't remember where door is. Really want to wash hands after touching *something* on toilet floor. But don't know where the wash-hand basin is. Touching walls. Found door, I think. Hard to tell with these modern buildings. Can't find door handle. ***Where is door handle?*** This what it must be like to be blind.... Awful.... So awful...... This is how my cat must have felt, when I was little, and my parents asked me to take it to the vet in a cardboard box with a handle. And the poor creature went crazy and clawed its way out as I wal-ked down our road. Awful..... Is there a door handle that's high up, or a low-down-slidey-one? **Oh God!** I *really hate* these rooms with no windows. I'm remembering when I got stuck in a lift and the light went out, and I was so frightened I almost passed out. There were two people with me that day. I'm alone now. This thought makes me panic a little. *I must NOT pass out with fright.* Tap on door with fingernails, and call out – not too loudly, because I feel embarrassed, and I don't want to sound like a silly hysterical female – but loud enough for someone passing by to hear me. This floor of the building seems very quiet and deserted, so I could have a *long* time to wait. Although someone may enter the waiting area nearby soon. *Hopefully.* Need to get out now because it's soon time for my appointment, and I've got three flights of stairs to climb, with rests on chairs at the top of each staircase for tired people like me..... *'HELLO! Can you let me out please? ...... Can't find door handle!'* ...... I wait.......... Ten seconds feels like ten hours......... Twenty seconds feels like twenty-thousand years.

2.06 p.m.    OH... NO!... I *really need* to sit down. I can't stand standing any longer..... can't stand it in here either, it's so *suffocatingly* pitch black. I will not pass out, *deep breath.... deep breath.... deep breath.* I don't recall seeing a chair when I first came into the room and the bloomin' light was still on. Suddenly feel very exhausted. Will have to sit on the floor, can't face going back into tiny toilet cubicle..... Floor is so *cold.* I'm feeling cold now..... *cough, cough, cough...* Someone may hear me coughing and check if I'm OK. But I very much doubt it...... *cough...... cough, cough.* They will probably think I'm having a crafty cigarette. **Is this really happening?** I'm going to *miss* my appointment. Could take *months* and *months* to get another one. Could take ages for Ben to find a parking space, and come and rescue me. Or he may be involved in an accident and end up in hospital for days. And I won't know what's happened to him. And. Why?.... *Why?*..... Why did I leave my mobile phone at home? And the lovely lady I've come to see will just think I've missed my appointment. That I've not turned up. And I've not bothered to let the clinic know there's been a problem. Feel so thirsty.... dry throat. Need drink of water, but no energy to crawl around room looking for wash-hand basin, and anyway I may put my hand in something soft and damp again...... Must be awful, being kidnapped and kept in the dark – cold, hungry and thirsty. Hungry now. **Oh God!** Have touched my face with the hand that touched something damp on the toilet floor – germs are going to be crawling into my mouth...... Ugh........ *Argh!* Something has just crawled over my hand. Am I going to die here? Will I soon be covered in cobwebs? I've come to a health clinic and it's going to kill me. I want to laugh.... Am I going mad? Must get up and tap on door again, if it is the door.

2.09 p.m.    *HELLO!... HELP!... Can somebody open the door please?*

ME:    OH, *thank goodness* you're back!.... Light went out. Couldn't see a thing..... **Pitch black**. Couldn't find door handles. So cold. I've been in here for *YEARS*. Have I gone grey? Must wash hands! Can you find the light switch? *Must wash hands!*

BEN:    You're safe now dear.

3.05 p.m.

BEN:      How was the healing treatment?

ME:      Wonderful.... So relaxing.... Feel sleepy.

BEN:      Not far to walk to the car.

ME:      You *actually found* a space fairly close to the clinic?

BEN:      Yeah. Miracles do 'appen!

* * * * * * * *

5.00 p.m.

BEN:      Nearly home. You look happy.

ME:      Can't believe how I'm feeling.

BEN:      The sparkle is back in your eye.

ME:      My head feels light and bright, like a white balloon, instead of a lump of black coal – no jokes about being an air head!

BEN:      Wouldn't dream of it dear.

ME:      Positive thoughts are popping into my head.

BEN:      Don't pop your white balloon.

ME:      I'm thinking about the countless photos I've taken of the view out of our bedroom window. Some came out really well – though I say it myself!

BEN: Don't become too inflated dear.

ME: I won't! But I will print out some of the photos, pop them in a clip frame, then put them on the wall either side of the window – the wonderful sunsets, rainbows, and snowy scenes. And there's some that will make you smile, because it's a chore you don't have to do anymore.

BEN: What's that?

ME: Scraping snow and ice off your car windows, very early on winter mornings.

BEN: Oh, yeah. Something I'm not going to miss.

ME: When I look at the photos I'll think how *bloomin' lucky* I was to have *a view* for almost thirty years.

BEN: Always look on the bright side of life (whistling the Monty Python song again).

6.10 p.m.

ME: *OH! MY! GOD!*

BEN: You OK?

ME: I've just climbed the stairs without feeling like my body is made of concrete, and I'm carrying a rucksack full of house bricks on my back. I feel like I'm made of thin, light, flexible strong wire.

BEN: I'll try not to wind you up then.

WE LAUGH

## Thursday 6th

10.10 a.m.  I stand at the bedroom window, gently stroking Diamanda's warm silky fur. She purrs contentedly.

10.11 a.m.  We yawn a big wide yawn together, showing lots of shiny white fangs. We stretch together too, displaying nicely manicured claws – although mine are not like sharp little razors.

10.12 a.m.  I must clip the claws on the paws of my back legs. I noticed they needed a trim yesterday, they're getting so long, soon I'll be able to climb trees with the squirrels. Must find the nail scissors. Can't find them anywhere. Maybe I'll claw the furniture like Diamanda, to keep them in shape.

10.13 a.m.  Her ears are in happy-cat-position today. So are mine, because the building site is oddly quiet and peaceful.

10.14 a.m.  It's a cold, pale grey day. Black crows strut about. Not a white hard hat in sight. Silent as the rave. The rave where all the ravers have gone home exhausted up to their sweaty ears, the DJ has switched off the electrics, and there's just the memory of deafening, repetitive, mind-numbing noise.

10.16 a.m.  Diamanda and I are enjoying, not just the peace – the stillness of the house. On Tuesday the houseplants were trembling so much their little leaves looked terrified.

10.17 a.m.  I'm almost trembling with delight at feeling *so much* better after yesterday's healing treatment. And bubbling tiny bubbles – miniature Prosecco bubbles of excitement about a parcel. It arrived yesterday while we were out, so there was a sorry-we-missed-you card waiting on the doormat when we arrived home. Ben is going to pick it up from the parcel place later today. Can't wait – he said if it's what he thinks it is, it's an early Christmas present that will light up my eyes like a Christmas tree.

10.18 a.m.   I sip a minty tea.

10.19 a.m.   And smile beatifically.

*I sip a minty tea*
*And smile beatifically*
*My eyes will light up nice and bright*
*Just like a Christmas tree*

10.20 a.m.   Do I feel some more verse coming on?
No. Not today.

10.21 a.m.   But I have a sparkle in my eye. And will have a fairy light twinkle too, if the parcel is what Ben thinks it is. Starting to feel a little Christmassy again!

11.26 a.m.   Feeling a *little more* Christmassy, now that three early Christmas cards have arrived from a relative, an old friend, and our vet. The one from our vet is a colourful cartoon of cats and dogs. Five singing cats wearing Santa hats from a relative. And from an old friend, a rather different take on the twelve days of Christmas. I don't think the artist was confident enough to draw people. The eight maids a milking is a painting of a jolly brown cow, the nine ladies dancing – a flamingo dancing, the ten lords a leaping – a leaping unicorn, the eleven pipers piping – an elephant with musical notes trumpeting out of its trunk, and the twelve drummers drumming, just a drum with two sticks. But it's a happy card, all the creatures are smiling – the turtle dove, the French hen (there's only one of each bird), the calling bird, goose-a-laying, swan a swimming, and of course a partridge in a pear tree.

11.30 a.m.  Smiling at the card with the cats wearing Santa hats, while stroking Diamanda's satin soft head. As she rubs her muzzle against the corner of the card, I'm wondering if you can buy Santa hats for pets, with holes for their ears. I would not be surprised if you can these days.

* * * * * * * *

2.12 p.m.

BEN:  Got the early Christmas surprise for you.

ME:  Oh goody!

BEN:  Close your eyes.

ME:  OK.

BEN:  Tight shut?

ME:  Yes.

BEN:  Both eyes?

ME:  Yes (closing right eye).

BEN:  Hold out your paws.

ME:     OK (smiling).

BEN:    A bit further apart.

ME:     Ooh! It's *big* and *very long* and tubular. But feels light.

BEN:    I couldn't wait till Christmas to give it to you dear.

ME:     Oh, thanks (opening eyes). I'm intrigued. Haven't got a clue what it is. Looks *very well* bubble wrapped.

BEN:    I'll open it, you'll hurt your paws. Got nail scissors handy?

ME:     Can't find them. I'll get the kitchen scissors.

* * * * * * * *

BEN:    Here you are.

ME:     A blank canvas?

BEN:    Look on the other side.

ME:     WOW! Oh my goodness! I've never seen a painting by numbers like this! It's huge, and *extremely* detailed.

BEN:    Do you like it?

ME:     Well, looking at the little technicolour print of what it will look like when it's painted, *I LOVE IT!*

BEN:    I thought you would. It'll keep you quiet for weeks (smiling to himself). Here's all the little paint pots and two paint brushes.

ME:        Sweet. Beautiful rainbow colours. Lots of different
           blues and greens. Red and yellows. Purples and or-
           anges. Can you cut the plastic pots apart for me?
           They smell like acrylic paints, so I won't need any
           thinners. The canvas needs to be stretched on a
           wooden frame, it's very crinkly. It'll look great on a
           frame. Can't wait to get started, it'll be a BIG CHAL-
           LENGE! Can you sort it for me this weekend? Or
           tomorrow, if you're not busy?

BEN:       Certainly dear.


## Friday 7th

11.40 p.m.   Two more early Christmas cards arrived from friends.
             A black, white and silvery design of a Christmas tree.
             And a colourful painting entitled, *Christmas Village*
             – country cottages nestled in a snowy valley, choir
             boys singing outside the village church, and village
             children building a snowman next to a huge Christ-
             mas tree draped with lights (the scene sprinkled
             with silvery glitter).

11.50 p.m.   Inspired, I opened the old cardboard box full of
             Christmas decorations (Ben had brought down from
             the attic on 1st December, but so far I had only sat
             and looked at it), found the fairy lights, then draped
             them around the mirror over the fireplace in the
             sitting room. After arranging five Christmas cards
             on the mantelpiece, I flopped onto the sofa, nestling
             in the cushions, to watch today's Christmassy fantasy
             film, *The Perfect Christmas Village* – about a woman
             who is magically transported into her idea of the
             ideal Christmas village. During the adverts I wrote
             five Christmas cards, addressed the envelopes, then

stamped them with festive stamps.

2.10 p.m.   I sat and smiled at the small pile of envelopes, with a nice little sigh of achievement. The fairy lights twinkled with approval.

2.15 p.m.   Celebrity Weekly lay open on the coffee table. As I sleepily began to peruse the pages, Diamanda jumped up onto the table, then sat on the magazine and began cat perusing – oozing purrs.

2.16 p.m.   I gently stroked her silky black head, and thought how much she would love a decorated Christmas tree to decimate – merrily climbing up the branches and playfully knocking off the baubles, one by one. Then take great cat-like pleasure tearing off all the tinsel, and become entangled in the long, golden, sparkly snakes.

2.20 p.m.   Ben plodded in through the front door, looking pleased with himself. He'd bought another *round-tuit* in town. A bulging carrier bag of *round-tuits,* to do some decorating. Hopefully he will get around to it.

2.21 p.m.   As he plonked on the sitting room chair, taking the weight off his feet, Diamanda plonked onto the floor, putting the weight on her paws to greet him.

2.22 p.m.   The pages of Celebrity Weekly were free for me to peruse again. I was told to get inspiration with the stars' best buys. A photo of Rochelle Humes (who had successfully filled Holly Willoughby's fashionable shoes on *This Morning*), wowed in a rust roll neck, tucked into a check, cream and brown pencil skirt with little chocolate-button-like buttons.

2.23 p.m.    Turning the pages, I noticed all the stars wore delicious looking clothes. Butterscotch and toffee coloured, chunky knits. Coffee and biscuit coloured, corduroy skirts and suits. Custard yellow tops and dresses. And accessories in shades of cream, milk chocolate and plain chocolate.

2.25 p.m.    I'm truly, madly, mouth-wateringly aware of a tin of a selection of *very tasty* looking biscuits that Ben bought as a gift for our vet and his assistants. I will ask him to drop it round to the surgery *A. S. A. P.*

2.30 p.m.    If I carefully peel off the tape holding the lid down, then sample one, will they notice?

2.31 p.m.    Yes. There will be one section, not full to the top with biscuit.

2.32 p.m.    I could take the top biscuit off each section? Then seal the lid again?

2.33 p.m.    No. I will feel guilty and greedy, *and* if I have to go to the vet with Ben in the future, I will have guilty-greedy-person written all over my face.

2.35 p.m.    I write a wildlife-in-the-snow Christmas card for the vet with lovely-generous-person curly handwriting. Then another one with the same design for Pauline, who lives at the end of our street.

3.14 p.m.

ME:          Can you drop a Christmas card into our vet with the biccies, *soon as poss?*

BEN:         Yeah.

ME:    And I've written one for Pauline at number one, can you pop that into her on the way?

BEN:    OK.

ME:    Would have been nice to have had a Christmas tree this year but –

BEN:    Not a good idea with little-miss-naughty-paws (smiling at Diamanda).

ME:    I'll drape red and gold tinsel here and there, on shelves and the bookshelves.

BEN:    That will no doubt end up here and there on the floor.

ME:    For sparkly fun time!

\* \* \* \* \* \* \* \* \*

4.04 p.m.    Dozing with Diamanda.

4.06 p.m.    Demolition has stopped for the day.

4.07 p.m.    Dreamily peaceful and poetic.

*I doze with Diamanda*
*Demolition is no more*
*If I decorate with tinsel*
*It will end up on the floor*

4.10 p.m.    I watch Danny DeVito feuding with a friend over who has the best Christmas lights, in *Deck The Halls*. They end up resorting to desperate measures to outdo each other.

*Danny DeVito*
*Decks the halls*
*With desperate measures*
*And silvery balls*

6.10 p.m.

BEN: I dropped the card and biscuits into the vets.

ME: Thank God! I mean, oh good. Thanks.

BEN: Gave Pauline her card too. She was on her way into town, so we had a chat.

ME: I expect she is as *thrilled* as we are about the new housing development, and all the *noise*.

BEN: Yeah (laughing).

ME: If she were Jane Austen she'd say it was *most disagreeable*.

## Saturday 8th

ME: The noise from the building site was most entertaining at times this morning.

BEN: Really? (raised eyebrows).

ME: Yes (smiling) *most agreeable* (posh voice).

BEN: Do enlighten me *my dearest*.

ME: I was watching *Carry On Abroad*. Do you remember that film – where at the end there's a flood at the hotel, the building starts to crumble, and the holiday makers are running around panicking in their nightwear?

BEN:        Yeah.

ME:         Well, when the pillars started to crack and fall down, and the floors crumbled and crashed to the floor below, *our house* started shaking. And some of the crashing noises in the film coincided with the demolition noises on the building site. So –

BEN:        You felt like you were in the film.

ME:         Yes! I was really there. It was *so funny* when there was a loud bang outside, at *exactly* the same moment as a bed with a couple on it fell through the floor. And *then* there was a smashing sound, *really close* to our house, at the part where Sydney James walks through a glass door, thinking the glass hasn't been put in yet.

BEN:        I'm sorry I missed that exciting experience (feigned sad eyes).

ME:         The best bit –

BEN:        There was a best bit?

ME:         You should have been at home! At the end of the film, when the hotel was half demolished, and everyone was rushing about trying to escape, the caterpillar tracks on the building site came near to our house – so our walls shook more than usual, making the pictures rattle, and one fell, crashing onto the fireplace smashing the glass. *So dramatic!*

83

BEN:    I'll clear up the glass before you or Diamanda cut
        your paws.

ME:     Thanks! Did you know the word for caterpillar orig-
        inates from the French word chatepelose – hairy cat?

BEN:    Fascinating (on hands and knees in fireplace, swee-
        ping up broken glass).

* * * * * * * *

1.11 p.m.    Standing. Staring in bathroom mirror. Frowning at
             BIG red spot on the tip of my nose.

1.21 p.m.    Sitting. On sofa browsing through the jewellery cat-
             alogue, Pia.

1.22 p.m.    Smiling. I spot a pair of Christmassy earrings – little
             silver reindeer with shiny red enamel noses. Rudolf
             earrings. Must order for my niece for Christmas,
             she will *LOVE* 'em.

1.23 p.m.    Diamanda rests a paw on the *Feline Fancy Acces-
             sories* page. I think she would like the playful faux-
             fur pom-pom beanie (with black cat design)  to play
             with.

1.24 p.m.    I'm tempted by the fine filigree, silver cat pendant
             and cute kitten mittens.

1.25 p.m.    Diamanda flicks her long black tail when I turn the
             page, she hasn't finished admiring the stoneware
             Cat's Whiskers trinket dish, it would make a pretty
             snack bowl.

1.30 p.m.    As I flick through Celebrity Weekly, the beauty treatment Advent calendars catch my eye. They look good, until I see the cost – between forty-five and three hundred pounds!

1.31 p.m.     They no longer look so appealing.

1.32 p.m.     If I could afford it, I would be *most tempted* by the Body Shop calendar at forty-five pounds – lots of miniature Dani Deer bath, body and skin care. If I was a celebrity with *lots* of money, I would treat my nose to the Jo Malone calendar – twenty-four drawers of miniature scented candles and colognes. Then I'd feel guilty for spending so much money on an Advent calendar and give it away to a charity. But only after I'd opened all the little windows and enjoyed a *good long sniff* of *every* cologne. Then carefully closed them up again.

* * * * * * * *

ME:       What has no body and no nose?

BEN:      Dunno. What has no body and no nose?

ME:       Nobody knows.

BEN:      Very amusing dear. Want anything in town Rudolf?

ME:       It is a BIG red spot isn't it (covering nose with hand). I could do with some spot concealer from the Body Shop.

BEN:      OK.

ME:       And I know it's a week into December, but I'd like an Advent calendar, if there's any left in the shops.

BEN:     A posh one with chocolates in, or just card?

ME:      Hmm, just a cardboard one with a nice pic – Santa and his reindeer, or wildlife. Don't want to get more spots.

BEN:     I'll see if I can get one with a pic of Rudolf and his beautiful big red nose.

ME:      But (covering nose with a tissue) if there's only calendars left with chocolates in, then you'll have to get one of those – I'll have spot concealer from the Body Shop.

BEN:     So that at Christmas *no body nose* (pointing to nose) you have a spotty face.

* * * * * * * * *

2.00 p.m.   Diamanda and I curled up on the sofa to watch *The Christmas Calendar* – a romantic film about a struggling baker, Laura Bell Bundy, who receives a handmade Advent calendar from a secret admirer and the locals become obsessed with who sent it.

2.12 p.m.   Started writing a few more Christmas cards during the advents (I mean adverts).

2.30 p.m.   I daydream – an Advent calendar from a secret admirer is *so romantic*.

3.10 p.m.

BEN:     Is this OK?

ME:      Perfect.

BEN: I thought you'd like a snowy scene with woodland wildlife.

ME: Yes, lovely glittery bits too. And it's quite romantic that you know *exactly* what I like. Almost as romantic as an Advent calendar from a secret admirer.

BEN: I couldn't find a calendar with a picture of Rudolf with a big red nose.

ME: Like mine (lifting the tip of Diamanda's tail and hiding my nose under it, as we lie on the sofa).

BEN: The calendars that were left, with chocolates in, didn't have Christmassy pictures.

ME: Just as well. My willpower deserts me more and more as the years go by. I'm like Miranda.

BEN: My niece?

ME: No, Miranda on TV, in her sit-com *Miranda* – do you remember the Christmas special?

BEN: No.

ME: Well, she's a chocolate lover, and at the start of the episode it's the eve of Christmas Eve, and her little friend Stevie comes round to her flat. Together they excitedly open a window in her chocolate Advent calendar, but there's no chocolate. Stevie asks Miranda where the chocolate is, and her reply is so funny!

BEN: I can imagine dear.

ME: She asks – who can sit in a room all day when there's

little chocolates behind windows, and not remove them, eat them all, then close all the windows like nothing ever happened?

BEN: Sounds like you last Christmas.

ME: It was the Christmas before. We'd lost two dear old pets, and two dear old people that year, and you found me a chocolate Advent calendar with a picture of dear old Santa Claus. The little pieces of chocolate were creamy milk chocolate, and melted in my mouth like sunshine melting snow. Milk chocolate is more *more-ish* than plain, so you *have* to eat more.

BEN: And more.

ME: Chocolates are like cats, it's hard to have just one.

BEN: Diamanda is so crazy, galloping around the house and climbing up and down the curtains, she is like three cats. She fills the house with cat!

ME: Like I ended up filling my mouth with Advent calendar chocolate. Apart from being milk chocolate, the pieces were more desirable because of their shape. The Christmas cracker ones snapped beautifully when you bit the end – you shared some of them with me, do you remember?

BEN: No.

ME: Sometimes I got the middle bit, and sometimes you did, like a real cracker.

BEN: I'm sure it was great fun dear.

ME:    Anyway, if today's calendar had been a chocolate one, I'd have shared the first eight with you, because I can open *eight windows* today – one after the other! Then with good intention I'd have left all the other windows closed. But in the following days, if something made me sad or stressed, or if I saw something awful on a pet rescue, or vet programme, the little windows –

BEN:   Would be opened one by one and all the chocs eaten.

ME:    Would you like to open a window or two with me now?

BEN:   No, I won't spoil your fun.

ME:    Oh good. Did you get the spot concealer?

BEN:   Forgot. But I *did* remember – close your eyes, and open your paws, paw pads up.

ME:    OK (smiling).

BEN:   Paws further apart.

ME:    Oh, it's HUGE! Feels like a tray of twenty-four mince pies.

BEN:   Open eyes.

ME:    What is it?

BEN:   Don't you remember?

ME:    No.

BEN: Unwrap it and see.

ME: Goody, love surprises........... *Ooh, I think I know what it is!*...... Will open it when I'm in a creative mood, it'll be something to look forward to.

* * * * * * * *

4.05 p.m. Admiring woodland creatures in the snow in my admiral..... admire – I mean Advent calendar.

4.06 p.m. I wonder where the window is in this wonderful winter wonderland, with a little number **1** on it...... Ah, found it, a square window near the bunnies hopping in the snow..... *pick.... pick.... pick.... pick.....* *open at last!* A picture of a partridge in a pear tree.

4.07 p.m. *Pick........ pick........ picking* away at the rectangular window with a number **2**, next to robins in the snow, that opens to reveal a pile of presents – red, yellow and green gift-wrapped boxes, tied with a big purple bow.

4.08 p.m. It will soon be time to find the energy to wrap presents with jolly Christmassy paper, labelled with small Christmassy stickers, written with my best, tiniest, Christmassy writing.

4.09 p.m. Can't find the window with a number **3**. It must be camouflaged in an animal's coat, or something. Think I'll rest my eyes now – feeling a bit worn out with excitement.

5.10 p.m.

BEN: I've got my work's Christmas *do* tonight.

90

ME: I'd forgotten (yawning).

BEN: Shall I chop some veg for your dinner?

ME: Um, no thanks, I'll have hot mince pies with ice cream. Nice energy giving food, and one can be naughty at Christmas. Well, it's getting close to Christmas.

BEN: You say that at the beginning of October.

ME: I didn't think you'd be going to the Christmas *do*.

BEN: Nor did I. They invited me, even though I'm retired now. The girls invited us both.

ME: That's nice, I'd like to be up to going but –

BEN: I know.

ME: But, hey! I've got six more Advent windows to open, and I may open my surprise package. And there's that Harry Potter prequel on tonight, about magical animals in New York, set in the nineteen twenties – can't remember the title. Something like, *Magical Beasts And Where To Hunt For Them*, or *Magical Animals And How To Look For Them*. Oh, by the way, you should wear your reindeer shirt tonight.

BEN: Reindeer?

ME: The shirt I gave you last Christmas from Joe Browns catalogue. You liked it! The white one with little black reindeer leaping, galloping or standing majestically, all over it – with bright red antlers.

BEN:       Not bright red noses?

ME:        No (covering nose with a tissue). It will look *fantastic* with your best black trousers. I'll find it for you.

BEN:       Ah, got the title – *Fantastic Beasts And Where To Find Them!*

\* \* \* \* \* \* \* \* \*

6.35 p.m.    I'm searching for the number **3** on the Advent calendar........... Ahah! Finally found it on a reindeer's coat....... *pick*....... *pick*....... *pick*. A pretty pic of two golden bells tied with a red bow. Number **4** next. Where is it?...... Where?..... It's hiding from me.

6.36 p.m.    Here it is, on the snowman wearing a floppy, top hat – on his stripy blue and white scarf. *Pick......* *pick..... pick....* this one is difficult to open. *Pick.......* *pick.... pick.... pick.* Hurrah! A mince pie, decorated with a sprig of holly.

6.40 p.m.    I'm deep in thought as I devour a deep-filled mince pie. Will heat up two more later, and the vanilla ice cream will be useful if I burn my mouth on piping hot, sweet, fruity and spicy mincemeat filling. I almost always do.

6.42 p.m.    Still deep in thought – Ben looked *hot,* wearing his cool reindeer shirt, but I think the black reindeer with red antlers design would have looked better with turquoise or Christmas-tree-green hooves.

## Sunday 9th

8.45 a.m.   Got a sore tongue.

8.46 a.m.   Sipping lovely, chilled Scottish mineral water.

8.47 a.m.   Crunching cold wholemeal toast.

8.48 a.m.   Smiling because I have *four more* Advent calendar windows to open.

8.49 a.m.   *Five* windows, including today's! Or shall I open just three windows and leave numbers **8** and **9** until tomorrow, so that I'll have three windows to open on Monday. Decisions, decisions.

8.50 a.m.   *Sip... sip... sip. Crunch... crunch... crunch.* Number **8** is a long rectangular window, whereas most of the windows are square – and I'm intrigued to know what the picture will be. Will it be something long. A trumpet? A Christmas cracker? A chocolate log? A cucumber? A sausage dog? *Sip... sip...* A banana? A flute? An umbrella? A limo? *Crunch....... crunch.* Now I'm being silly. But it's the time of year to be silly – wear paper crowns, pull crackers, open funny gifts and have snowball fights.

8.51 a.m.   *Pick..... pick...* I open number **5** to find a snowflake. *Pick.... pick.... pick.....* number **6** is a rocking horse. *Pick.... pick.... pick.... pick....* number **7** makes me want to dip into the box of Christmas decorations again – it's a pic of a Christmas tree festooned with colourful baubles, topped with a star.

8.52 a.m.   Resisting opening number **8**, I will *pick* the right moment. It'll be something to look forward to.

8.53 a.m.    Think I'll continue decorating the sitting room today – hang festive decorations on the fairy lights around the fireplace mirror, away from small mischievous black and white paws. It's *SO VERY LOVELY* to have more energy since my appointment on Wednesday.

9.25 a.m.    I open number **8** – I resisted for thirty-three whole minutes. The rectangular window reveals a chocolate log, decorated with a robin, snowman and a Christmas tree. Sweet.

9.26 a.m.    I fancy nibbling something sweet now. A hot mince pie? No. A cold mince pie? No, they are much nicer hot. A banana will do. A *really ripe,* spreadable-soft, almost black banana, drizzled with honey – healthy without the high.

* * * * * * * *

10.45 a.m.    Head in freezer, searching for the veggie burgers, I spot a box of mince pies.

10.48 a.m.    Place two mince pies on a baking tray.

10.49 a.m.

ME:    I like the word *drizzled* don't you?

BEN:    Dunno.

ME:    When I lived with my parents, I used to love *drizzling* golden honey, fresh from the comb, onto freshly baked white bread that had been generously spread with thick, creamy, yummy-yellow Anchor butter.

BEN:    That's nice.

ME:     There's an advert on at the moment – chocolate being *drizzled* over something dark and divinely chocolatey. I can't remember what the advert is for, have you seen it?

BEN:    Yeah.

ME:     Can you remember what it's for?

BEN:    No.

ME:     Best of all, *drizzled* brings to mind perfectly cooked, beautifully artily arranged cuisine, in the centre of a square white plate, with a delicate sprig of herb and a tiny *drizzle* of sauce, in a colour that compliments the food - maybe crimson over a lime green terrine. Served with compliments of the head chef, as you sit at a table for two with a crisp white linen tablecloth, opposite a handsome man who showers you with compliments.

BEN:    And when you leave the restaurant – him, with an *empty* wallet – you feeling *full*, you both get wet because of the b***** *drizzle*, because you didn't bring an umbrella because the b***** weather man didn't mention wintry showers.

ME:     Fancy a mince pie with your coffee, Mr Cheerful?

BEN:    Yeah! (eyes lighting up like a Christmas tree).

ME:     One or two?

BEN:    Two (licking lips). You not having one?

ME:     Not today.

10.50 a.m.   I pop another pie on the baking tray.

BEN:        Changed your mind then?

ME:         The aroma of hot pie will be too tempting. I'll do a spot of little birdie watching to help me wait for the little pie to cool down – a little bit.

11.05 a.m.

ME:         There's a robin feeding on the bird table, isn't he delightful?

BEN:        Fery luffly – Ah, fery hot! (mouthful of mince pie).

ME:         The red feathers are beautiful. And he stands out, looking *so Christmassy* when it snows. I *love* the blue feathers too.

BEN:        Blue?

ME:         Have you ever *really* looked at a robin?

BEN:        No, not really.

ME:         The blue feathers are the loveliest soft-grey-blue, like a November sky. The brown feathers are the bare branches of trees in December. The white feathers, like fluffy snowflakes in January. The red feathers –

BEN:        Are like your nose when you get a cold in February, or you've got a spot right on the tip of –

ME:         I was *going to say* the rosy cheeks of children playing in the snow. Have a look at the robin, he's –

BEN:    Just flown off, you embarrassed him. And I'm off to Bill's in half an hour for a bracing walk on the beach, get some sea air in my feathers.

ME:     And burn off two-mince-pies-worth of calories.

\* \* \* \* \* \* \* \*

1.25 p.m.   Watching *Home Alone*.

1.26 p.m.   Will write a few Christmas cards during the ads.

1.43 p.m.   I sing along to *Rocking Around The Christmas Tree* with little Macaulay Culkin, as I drape tinsel around pictures on the wall.

1.50 p.m.   I'm flopped on the sofa, sleepily singing along to *White Christmas,* as I gently stroke warm, silky, black fur.

1.51 p.m.   Diamanda purrs.

3.45 p.m.   Softly singing to myself.

*Have yourself a merry little Christmas.*
*Tra, la la, la la.*

3.46 p.m.   As snowflakes fall at the end of the film, my eyelashes start to flutter.

3.47 p.m.   My eyes are closing *very slowly,* as I admire my neat little pile of Christmas cards.

3.48 p.m.   I'm dreaming of a white Christmas.

## Monday 10th

8.00 a.m.   *CRASH! CRASH!... rumble.... rumble.... rumble.....  dig..... dig...... dig.* The excavation and demolition monsters have come back to life after their day of rest.

8.30 a.m.   *Pick.... pick.... pick.* I open window number **10** to find a robin in the snow.

8.31 a.m.   I daydream of a white Christmas. The building site will look so much better covered with a crispy, white blanket.

8.32 a.m.   My heart feels a little sad. I will no longer be able to sit and enjoy watching children building snowmen in the car park, throwing snowballs and shrieking with delight. Must get a *round-tuit* and frame a photo I took of children playing in the snow, to put on our wall.

10.10 a.m.   A hand delivered Christmas card is gently slipped through our letter box and flops onto the mat.

10.12 a.m.   My heart is up-lifted when I open it. I don't *believe it!* It's a delightful painting of children in the snow, wearing woolly bobble hats, scarves and mittens, and building a snowman! I will sit it in the window. It's from a dear old lady who used to live next door to us a few years ago. No doubt, when she saw the goings-on in the what-used-to-be-a-car park, she felt relieved that she had moved house. Must check my pile of cards to see if I have written one for her.

10.13 a.m.   Yes! Envelope addressed and stamped. I'm tempted to open the envelope and write a message in her card, saying I thought she must feel *very* happy *and* relieved that she has moved away now.

10.30 a.m.   I must dig last week's TV Weekly out of the recycling bag to read what happened in Friday's episode of *Coronation Street*. I forgot to watch the repeats at the weekend – my mind full of Christmas thoughts and mouth full of mince pie. The programme can become a little boring if you start to miss episodes, storylines change so quickly these days. Or maybe it's me, my brain slowing down over the years, and my memory quickly forgetting what's going on. Who is angry with whom? Who is going to make it right? Who has got themselves into a right pickle? Who thinks they are right when they are so very wrong? Who is secretly planning revenge? Who is falling in love? Who is falling out of love? Who is in prison? Who will soon be out of prison?....

10.35 a.m.   Hurrah! Found last week's TV Weekly. Now have an idea about some of what's going on. Eileen enjoys an unexpected windfall and her friends recommend a holiday, so I expect we'll see her on holiday in a future episode. Sinead makes a disturbing discovery – hope I find out what it was. And there's more acrimony between Nick and Carla – no surprise there.

1.05 p.m.   I can actually hear the women talking on *Loose Women*, now that the workmen outside have gone for their lunch break.

1.20 p.m.   Another Christmas card appears through the letter box, hand delivered from Pauline at number 1.

1.21 p.m.   Have I written one to her?...... Yes. Ben delivered it last week. Wish I had written a little message about

about the new housing estate, apart from wishing her a lovely Christmas – from what Ben said, I know she feels the same way as us, about the noise, saucepans rattling on her cooker, and the fillings rattling in her teeth.

1.34 p.m.    I show Ben the Christmas card from Pauline.

ME:    Notice the blue feathers on the robin?

BEN:    Oh yeah.

2.10 p.m.    The romantic drama, *A Snow White Christmas* is on TV. I write the last of the Christmas cards and letters during the adverts.

ME:    I'm dreaming of a white Christmas.

BEN:    I'm getting a *round-tuit,* so you'll have snow white paintwork on the kitchen ceiling today.

ME:    You're painting? (hand on forehead) Wonders will never cease!

BEN:    Have you opened your surprise parcel yet?

ME:    No, I'm saving it. It's something to look forward to. I've had Christmas cards and letters to write, to keep me occupied.

BEN:    Shall I post those cards for you?

ME:    Not just yet, I'm enjoying gazing at the beautiful big pile – a job well done.

BEN:    Who sent the card with the children wearing bobble

hats in the snow?

ME: It's from Jean, who used to live next door.

BEN: That's nice.

ME: Did you know French sailors used to wear bobble hats to protect their heads?

BEN: From snowballs?

ME: No, the low, wooden beams on ships.

BEN: Fascinating dear.

## Tuesday 11th

8.20 a.m. Bunnies were hopping around in the snow today, in window number **11**. They were so delightful that I wanted to open another window.

8.21 a.m. But I decided to be good and wait until tomorrow, and just enjoy a daydream about frolicking in the snow with bunnies.

8.22 a.m. Diamanda had other ideas. She sat on the calendar so I couldn't move it, then started picking at number **24** with her beautifully newly-sharpened-on-the-side-of-the-sofa claw. She was much better at *pick.... pick.... picking....* than me. I told her she should wait until Christmas Eve to open that window, and gently tried to deter her. But of course, being a cat, this made her even more determined. Maybe she thought there would be a mouse in the hay of a cradle, in a stable in Bethlehem...... I smiled...... Then gave up.

8.23 a.m.    Diamanda lost interest with the almost-half-open window, so I closed it up quickly before I was tempted to have a sneaky peek. Then she started picking away at number **14** and number **18**. *Pick... pick... pick... purr... purr... purr* – and having so much fun, I let her carry on.

8.24 a.m.    Of course, now that I wasn't bothered, Diamanda lost interest and headed for the bedroom window to see what the workmen were up to today. The corner of window number **14** was open only a tiny bit, so it was easy to close up, but number **18** was half open and I couldn't resist a quick glance. It looked like a deer in the snow.

8.26 a.m.    *I didn't see it. I didn't see the deer in the snow.* I'm erasing it from my mind already, like an eager school-girl with a new pencil rubber, removing a big mistake – a *BIG* mistake, like her ex-boyfriend. What *did she see in him?!* What *was she thinking?*

8.27 a.m.    I'll have forgotten by the 18<sup>th</sup> anyway.

10.10 a.m.    Leisurely leafing through ACE catalogue Christmas bargains, I notice something I would *love* in the children's section – a unicorn with moving eyes, mouth and a horn that lights up for (the catalogue says) a mystical effect.

10.11 a.m.    Diamanda appears out of nowhere and glances at me with big, bright eyes. Then licks her whiskery mouth with an *is-there-tuna* tongue, to remind me that I already have a mystical creature, and she *does not* want another one in the house.

10.12 a.m.    I would like the Seven Dwarves Christmas tree decorations – if we had a tree this year. But we have a little black mystical creature with half feral paws and climb-loving claws, that feel the feline need to bat anything that dangles or could be rolled around on the carpet.

10.13 a.m.   Diamanda twitches the end of her tail to let me know she isn't bothered, as she pads past me, head held high, with an air of *I'm-the-queen-of-this-house.*

10.14 a.m.   Turning the pages, I spot a bright yellow ride-on pedal digger and bright red tractor for children. There's a ride-on JCB excavator/digger with bucket scoop, complete with detachable trailer and hard hat too.

10.16 a.m.   The building site is deserted today.

10.17 a.m.   Oh! How I would *love to* ride up and down the mounds of earth on a battery operated children's tractor, wearing a little yellow hard hat.

11.10 a.m.   Sipping de-caf coffee (riding up and down mounds of earth in my mind's eye).

11.11 a.m.   Crunching honey spread on toast.

11.12 a.m.   Perusing double page spread about the Royal family's Christmas in Weekly Wife.

11.34 a.m.

ME:   Want to hear about the Royal Family's Christmas?

BEN:   No, not really, but I'm sure you're going to tell me.

ME:        I'll spare you the details about the gathering of family at Sandringham House in Norfolk on Christmas Eve. And the tradition of when and where they open their presents, and the church service on Christmas Day.

BEN:     Lucky me.

ME:        But I was interested to know the Queen gives her staff a book or gift token to the value of thirty-five pounds and a Christmas pudding. While the puds used to come from Fortnum and Mason, today she apparently buys Tesco's finest.

BEN:     Lucky Tesco.

ME:        Last year was Meghan's first Christmas with the Royal Family. And hearing of the Queen's penchant for gift jokes, the more ridiculous the better, she decided to buy her a singing toy hamster. And guess what?

BEN:     I've no idea.

ME:        The Queen loved it!

BEN:     My Christmas will be *so much happier* now that you have shared that marvellous piece of information with me dear.

## Wednesday 12th

8.46 a.m.

ME:        *Delicious!* I love freshly laid boiled eggs from happy hens on toast.

BEN: The hens are happy perching on toast are they?

ME: Well, you never know, they may like something toasty warm to lay their eggs on.

BEN: Rob said his *girls* are laying again.

ME: Sweet, I love it that he calls his hens, his girls. And so kind of him to give us a box. I like the odd bit of straw stuck to the eggs, you don't get *that* from Sainsbury's free range.

BEN: Yeah (munch, munch).

ME: Would you believe today's Advent calendar window is a picture of three French hens!

BEN: How do you know they are French?

ME: Well, they must be, remember the Christmas song?

> *Four calling birds*
> *Three French hens*
> *Two turtle doves*
> *And a partridge in a pear tree*

BEN: Oh, yeah (munch, munch).

ME: My parents grew pear trees. I wish I'd put a toy partridge in one of them at Christmas – would've been a laugh.

BEN: Hilarious (slurp, slurp).

ME: The house is shaking so much this morning, if we had a Christmas tree, the decorations would be swinging madly from side to side. If we had the Seven Dwarves decorations, they would appear to be dancing.

BEN: Yeah (munch, munch).

ME: I'd like a child's tractor to ride up and down the mounds of earth on the building site. It would be fun.

BEN: Doesn't surprise me (munch, munch).

ME: You can get little JCB's with diggers for children too, aren't they sweet? (pointing to a page in ACE catalogue). I could have a great time when the workmen have gone home for the day.

BEN: You could watch some mountain climbing instead. The film *Everest* is on tonight, about two mountain climbing expeditions.

ME: A film about me would be entitled *Forever Rest!* (turning the catalogue page).

BEN: I expect you'd like that pink unicorn with light up horn too.

ME: Oh, I hadn't noticed it.

BEN: Really? (smiling with raised eyebrows). Opened your parcel yet?

ME: I'll get all the prezzies wrapped, and finish making the sitting room Christmassy first. If it's what I think it is, it'll be quite a big project and take a *lot of effort* and concentration.

BEN:     Keep you quiet for weeks.

ME:      Maybe months.

BEN:     Even better.

\* \* \* \* \* \* \* \*

ME:      I don't think I can watch *Coronation Street* tonight.

BEN:     Why?

ME:      The Sinead and Daniel storyline is too sad, Monday's episode had me in floods.

BEN:     What are you like.

ME:      I'll watch that rom-com about two women exchanging houses opposite sides of the Atlantic over Christmas – *The Holiday*, with Kate Winslet, Cameron Diaz and an actor whose name I can never remember. You've seen the film, can you remember his name?

BEN:     No idea.

ME:      There's a couple Christmas dramas on today – *The Christmas Gift* and *Twelve days of giving*. I will wrap prezzies and watch *The Christmas gift*.

BEN:     Splendid idea.

## Thursday 13th

Another Christmas card arrived today – an arty black and white photo of a stag in the snow, from my sister and family.

Beautiful. I placed it in the window, next to the card with a picture of children building a snowman, bunnies frolicking in the snow, and a snowy Christmas village scene.

   Today's Advent window opened to reveal a pile of Christmas presents. I made a mental note – must wrap more gifts. Then I sat admiring the festive cards and wishing it would snow.

* * * * * * * *

1.01 p.m.  We received sad news about a relative passing away.

1.05 p.m.  But life must go on.

1.08 p.m.  We must continue to send good cheer.

1.09 p.m.  Do Christmassy things.

1.10 p.m.  Eat. Wash. Watch TV. Sleep.

1.11 p.m.  When all you want to do is sit in silence.

1.12 p.m.  Feed the cat. Stroke the cat.

1.13 p.m.  Keep getting a *round-tuit*.

1.14 p.m.  Even though your energy has deserted you.

1.15 p.m.  And you feel you will never move again.

1.16 p.m.  Never smile again.

1.17 p.m.  Ever.

1.18 p.m.  But you put on a brave face.

| | |
|---|---|
| 1.20 p.m. | Laugh at little things. |
| 1.21 p.m. | When all you want to do is cry. |
| 1.22 p.m. | Cry your heart out. |
| 1.23 p.m. | Why are sad things sadder at Christmas? |
| 1.24 p.m. | I suppose it's obvious really. |

* * * * * * * *

2.04 p.m.    There's a joyful song on an advert on TV.

> *It's the most wonderful time of the year*
> *With the kids jingle belling*
> *And everyone telling you 'Be of good cheer'*
> *It's the most wonderful time of the year*

2.07 p.m.    Singing quietly to self while draping tinsel on a shelf.

> *It can be the most miserable time of the year*
> *Decorating a tree when you've no energy*
> *La la, la la, la!*

2.15 p.m.    Two young children are arguing loudly outside our house.

> *It's the most miserable time of the year*
> *Lots of cards need-a-writing*
> *And kids won't stop fighting*
> *La la, la la, la!*

2.40 p.m.    Wrapping a few presents with bright red, green, and silver mistletoe design, cheers me up a little.

*It's the most wonderful time of the year*
*There'll be much mistletoeing*
*And hearts will be glowing when loved ones are*
*near*
*It's the most wonderful time of the year*

3.15 p.m.    Watching the cartoon version of *A Christmas Carol* lightens my sprouts – I mean spirits.

*It's the most wonderful time of the year*
*There'll be scary ghost stories*
*And tales of the glories of la la la la!*

4.35 p.m.    I doze off with Diamanda to dream of a winter wonderland, where the jolly Ghost of Christmas Present hands out presents to wildlife in a forest. A robin, two turtle doves and three French hens, sing festive melodies, perched on snowy branches. Squirrels nibble sprouts and chestnuts. Tiny snowflakes fall as Kate Winslet and Cameron Diaz feed mince pies to the deer. The Seven Dwarves appear on mini tractors and build a snowman with Snow White. And all the fun is watched by the comedian Alan Partridge as he sits in a pear tree.

5.20 p.m.

BEN:    I'm off to Sainsbury's in a minute for some beers, thought I'd get us a treat for dinner, what do you fancy?

ME:    There was a little bird in the garden today that sounded like it was singing *pizza, pizza, pizza....* *pizza, pizza, pizza....* so I fancy –

BEN:    There's one in the freezer.

ME:         The thin 'n' crispy? Topped with tomato sauce and mozzarella, cheddar, grilled red 'n' yellow peppers, onion and spinach and pesto drizzle – love the word *drizzle* – flavoured with garlic, marjoram, thyme, oregano, basil and lots of things I should be avoiding?

BEN:      That's the one!

ME:         Lovely. Oh, and there was a little bird that chirruped, *chip, chip, chip*....... *chip, chip, chip*...... I can hear it now, listen. Can you hear it?

BEN:      Yeah!...... Is that another little bird I can hear singing, *salad, salad, salad*?

ME:         Very amusing dear. I don't fancy lettuce, cucumber or tomatoes, but I can hear a crow – *caw, caw, coleslaw*..... *caw, caw, coleslaw*.

BEN:      That's dinner sorted then.

ME:         *Love Actually* is on tonight, I'm going to get very weepy so –

BEN:      You'll be needing a box of Kleenex and a nice bottle of wine to go with dinner? And maybe a sweet treat for afters?

ME:         Sounds *perfetto*.

> *It's the most wonderful time of the year*
> *There'll be pizza and wine*
> *And the church bells will chime*
> *La la, la la la la!*

## Friday 14th

9.00 a.m.

ME: I woke up in a strange position today, I usually wake up on my side. Today I was on my back with my left hand on my hip and my right arm lifted – a sort of teapot position. Weird.

BEN: Maybe you need to *pour out* your feelings dear.

ME: Well, I had a lovely weep watching *Love Actually* last night, so maybe I just feel something *brewing*.

BEN: A storm?

ME: It'll be just a storm in a teacup.

BEN: I'll make us a brew, as the Northerners say...... Oh, I see you've just had a coffee so –

ME: That would be *lovely actually*.

BEN: Do you want me to take the Christmas cards and parcels to the post office today?

ME: Not quite finished parcelling up yet, I need to get a *round-tuit*.

BEN: I'll get you a *round-tuit* in town, they are going cheap in Wilko at the moment.

ME: Oh thanks, that's handy!

9.05 a.m. I softly sing some lyrics of a song by The Beach Boys, changing the words a little.

*Round round, get around*
*I get around*
*I get a round-tuit*
*I get around*

*I get around*
*la la, la la la*
*On my witches broom*
*Like a rocket zoom*

BEN: I haven't seen those salt and pepper pots before.

ME: Salt and pepper pots?

BEN: The white china ones on the kitchen drainer.

ME: Oh, we've had them for about twenty-five years, I found them in the cellar covered in dust – a Christmas present from a relative I think. Sweet aren't they. I like the curly tails and pointy mouse noses – cleaned up well after a good wash.

BEN: Are they *squeaky* clean?

ME: Very!

BEN: How long will it be before Diamanda knocks them onto the floor and plays with them?

ME: Not long.

BEN: What *are* you doing?

ME: I'm crumbling up the pastry from a mince pie – a festive treat for our robin. I've noticed robins seem to enjoy pastry or bread more than the peanuts, unlike the other birds.

BEN:      That's interesting dear.

ME:      And I read in Weekly Wife, according to tradition, a bride woken by a robin on her big day will be eternally blessed, isn't that nice.

BEN:      Yeah, very nice.

ME:      I also read, studies show the UK consumes an average of three hundred million mince pies every Christmas!

BEN:      Fascinating.

ME:      Shall I? (pointing to the last two mince pies and turning the oven on).

BEN:      Yep (licking lips in anticipation).

ME:      We will eat two of the three hundred million devoured in the UK.

* * * * * * * *

10.05 a.m. Diamanda and I watch a robin, and a pair of blue tits pecking happily on the bird table.

10.06 a.m. I think – *how delightful.*

10.07 a.m. Diamanda thinks – *how delicious.*

10.08 a.m. The robin feeds on the mince pie crumbs. The blue tits feed on the peanuts.

ME:      The robins prefer pastry to peanuts – look!

BEN:     That's a nice little pair of tits.

ME:      Yes dear.

BEN:     Why do women have big boobs?

ME:      Well, I imagine the answer isn't, so they can feed their babies with lots of nutritious breast milk. So, tell me why do women have big boobs?

BEN:     So men have something to look at while they are talking.

ME:      Men!...... Oh, can you get soya milk when you're in town. And something else.... can't remember.

BEN:     You'll remember as soon as I've gone out of the door. Text me.

ME:      OK.

* * * * * * * *

1.25 p.m.

BEN:     Here you are, soya milk and mince pies madam.

ME:      Thank you kind sir.

BEN:     You look very festive in your navy jumper, with white snowflakes all over it.

ME:      Lovely isn't it, like snowflakes in the night! I wish they were *real* snowflakes. There was a little Christmas jumper in my Advent calendar window today – reminded me it's Christmas Jumper Day.

BEN:     Is it?

ME:     You should have one.

BEN:     A mince pie or a jumper? (opening the box of mince pies).

ME:     You'd look good in a jumper with a Christmas pudding design. A lovely round pudding on your nicely rounded belly.

BEN:     I have a new spiky hair cut, that could be the sprig of holly on top!

ME:     I could dye it green for you. And you could wear a red berry earring – be good practice for the next Faerie Festival we go to.

BEN:     Anything you say dear.

* * * * * * * *

1.45 p.m.     As work continues opposite our house (rocks rolling down mounds of rubble, and the house shaking), I watch the Christmas decorations I've dangled on the fairy lights (a rocking horse, trumpet, star, angel, snowman and a snowflake) gently sway to the music of mayhem, and wonder whether to watch the romantic film, *Rock and Roll Christmas* or a nice family film, *Let it Snow*.

1.50 p.m.     I switch the kettle on for a warming cuppa, ready to curl up with Diamanda to watch *Let it Snow*.

116

1.52 p.m.     I draw a snowflake with my forefinger in the condensation on the kitchen window.

1.53 p.m.     And wish for snow.

## Saturday 15th

This morning the sky was pale winter-blue with
streaky clouds, like angel wings, as I shivered my way to the bird
table, wearing my fluffy, white slipper boots and dressing gown,
like a weary snowman plodding down the garden. The breeze
felt icy-snowman-cold on my pink-womanly-warm face.

The collared doves, as always, were first to descend
onto the bird table. Then a single white dove appeared, and I felt
*very peaceful*. Our beautiful, bright red-breasted robin bobbed
nearby on the fence, followed by one of our squirrels bounding
down from a sycamore tree, tail quivering, beady eyes eager for
her morning feast. I felt *very poetic*. Then I noticed a bird had
done its business down our kitchen window pane, and wondered when I'd have the energy to clean it off. I stopped feeling
*peaceful* and *poetic*, and tried not to feel like *pooh*. But only for
a moment, because I remembered my dreams, and a little smile
spread across my face, like butter on a thick slice of hot, toasted
wholemeal bread – warming my mind.

A few sheep had wandered into our garden to graze
on the lawn, followed by shepherds watching their flocks and
three wise men. I've no doubt my dream was inspired by the
nativity scene in *The Vicar of Dibley,* I had watched just before
bedtime. I'm surprised I didn't dream of finding the baby Jesus
wrapped in swaddling tea towels in the kitchen sink, who had to
be rescued by me so that the shepherds could wash their socks
by night.

Today's Advent calendar window (that curious claws
had started to open) opened to reveal a snowman with a carrot
nose, coal for his eyes, tree branches for arms, and a woolly red

scarf.

After opening the Advent window, I closed the kitchen window, then gazed at the sky, deep in thought... please let it snow.... a deeply deep, beautiful white blanket of snow.... deep and *crisp* and *even,* like a deep pan, *crisp* and *even* pizza. It makes this time of year so much more magical. And we all need a little sparkle in our lives.

Loads of Christmas cards poured through the letter box. Well, four *really*. But they felt like a nice little pile to open. There was a nativity scene, which inspired me to sing.

> *While shepherds wash their socks by night*
> *All watching ITV*
> *The angel of the Lord came down and*
> *Turned to BBC*

The other cards were silvery, glittery snowflakes on a black background, choir boys singing in the snow, and a mouth painting of angels – all delightful artworks that inspired me to doodle little snowflakes flying around with angels, on the back of an envelope.

I arranged the cards on the coffee table and sat back to admire my small art collection. Then Diamanda appeared, leapt onto the table, knocked the cards over, one by one, then sat where I could admire her fabulous feline body instead. I stroked her head, complimenting her on her bright eyes and fine whiskers. She purred and I recalled a saying by Leonardo da Vinci.

> *The smallest feline is a masterpiece.*

BEN:      It's getting very chilly now (plodding in through the front door, and into the kitchen).

ME:      Hot coffee and a hot mince pie?

BEN:     Two please!

ME:      I'll turn the oven on.

BEN:     I'll turn the heating up........ What *are* you doing?

ME:      I'm feeling a little chilly (stroking a red chilli pepper).

BEN:     What are you like.

* * * * * * * *

ME:      The condensation in the corners of the windows looks a bit like snow.

BEN:     Wishful thinking.

ME:      Arctic foxes have special blood vessels in their paws that circulate the blood twice as fast, so their feet don't get cold.

BEN:     Clever foxes. I expect you'll be watching *Cold Feet* tonight.

ME:      I will (nose in TV Weekly). And I'm looking forward to more Christmas TV – *The Polar Express, White Christmas* and *Frozen*.

BEN:     You will have Christmas square eyes.

ME:      And you will have a Christmas round belly!

* * * * * * * *

BEN:     Are there any Christmas cards left?

ME:      Yes, lots. Robins in the snow. Foxes, hedgehogs, owls, deer, squirrels in the snow –

BEN:     Did you know squirrels grow their brains a bit in Autumn?

ME:      Really? Is this a joke?

BEN:     No, it's so they can map where their stashes are. Saw it on a nature programme.

ME:      Clever squirrels!....... Anyway, we've got cards with wildlife in the snow or just snow.

BEN:     Just snow?

ME:      A garden in the snow.

BEN:     I'll let you decide.

ME:      How many do you need?

BEN:     Just the one. Got any stamps left?

ME:      One first class and one second. One second?

BEN:     Both.

ME:      Both?

BEN:     I'm sending a card to Hungary. It'll cost exactly one first and one second. Can you write it in your nice handwriting?

ME:      Will do. Give me just *one second*.

BEN:     Very amusing dear.

ME:      Who am I writing the card to?

BEN:     Adam and Meli, spelt M, e, l, i.

ME:      If your name was Adam I'd be tempted to change my name to Evie.

BEN:     And you'd name our house Eden.

ME:      I would.......... A Christmas cracker joke springs to mind! What did Adam say on the day before Christmas?

BEN:     No idea. What did Adam say on the day before Christmas?

ME:      It's Christmas, Eve!

BEN:     Good one (smiling).

ME:      I'll send Adam and Evie, I mean Meli, a card with a photo of a garden in the snow.

*I'm dreaming of a white Christmas*
*With every Christmas card I write*

*May your days be merry and bright*
*And may all your Christmases be -*

BEN:     Look out of the window.

ME:      Must I?

BEN:     Yeah.

ME:      Can't you just tell me.

BEN:     No.

ME:      I'm too tired to move.

BEN:     It'll make you smile.

ME:      I'll look in a minute or a two.

BEN:     You should look now.

ME:      Is it that huge fox?

BEN:     No.

ME:      The little bird that's rarely seen in our part of the country?

BEN:     No, have another guess.

ME:      The black cat with the very long tail, that looks like a panther?

BEN:     It's something white.

ME:      The beautiful fluffy white cat?

BEN:     It's something *white and fluffy*.

ME:      It's not? (eyes lighting up).

BEN:     Yeah, what you've been dreaming of.

ME:      Is it settling?

BEN:        It is.

ME:         Ooh, I must see!

* * * * * * * *

*How full of the creative genius is the air in which these are generated! I should hardly admire more if real stars fell and lodged on my coat.*

Henry David Thoreau

# January

## Monday 7th

7.25 p.m.

ME:       *Ooh, lovely!* That's better (flopping into a large, soft and very comfy sofa in front of an inglenook fireplace, the roaring log fire warming my cold nose). That was my exercise for the week!

BEN:     Exercise?

ME:       Yes! In my stars, Cosmic Colin said exercise is ideal to keep me calm and focused this week. I've just walked about ten steps from our front door to our car. Then plodded about another twenty-five steps from the car, into the pub, then to the bar. Then stood at the bar trying to look like a normal customer and not someone who wants to tell the barman that if he doesn't serve me soon I will most certainly collapse on the nicely polished floor *and* if I do he will panic because he looks *SO* young *and* he won't know what to do because this situation wasn't in his training and I will feel *SO* embarrassed for embarrassing him and –

BEN:     And you've plodded another nine or ten steps to the sofa. Then –

ME:       Flop!

BEN:     Like an egg in flour.

ME:       In front of a *LOVELY,* deliciously warm fire. The heat making my spirits lift, like a Victoria sponge cake on

125

gas mark six.

\* \* \* \* \* \* \* \*

BEN: What did my stars say?

ME: Can't remember..... *sip*...... *sip*....... Ah, the bubbles are going to my head and waking up my brain. Colin said, when you are setting your targets for the new year ahead, include creative activities. You've been practising songs on your guitar for gigs, so you're heading in the right direction. And you mustn't forget, decorating your home, making it look beautiful, can be creative.

BEN: Yes dear...... *sip*...... *sip*....... I'll remember that.

ME: Belated happy New Year! (raising glass).

BEN: Happy New Year!

ME: You're a lot slimmer than this time last year, so I should say happy new *rear*.

*You are my rear of the year*
*That is very plainly clear*

BEN: *Thank you, thank you*
*Thank you, thank you*
*Thank you so much dear.*

ME: You're welcome.

BEN: Flattery will get you everywhere.

ME: Will it get you up the stairs to paint the stair wall?

BEN: I doubt it.

ME: There's no harm in trying, everyone needs a little encouragement sometimes – you do get rather *behind*
with the DIY.

BEN: Here's to going forward (raising glass). Bottoms up!

\* \* \* \* \* \* \* \*

ME: I should've taken the Christmas cards and decorations down at he weekend.

BEN: Yeah.

ME: But they look so sparkly.... *sip*.... *sip*.... and twinkly,
colourful and cheery, when in winter, life can be so
dreary.

BEN: Do you feel more verse coming on?

ME: *He toasts the new yeary*
*With eyes a little bleary*
*Drinking half a pint of beery*

BEN: *She feels a little weary*
*Because life can be so dreary*

ME: *Then he sniffs, a little teary*

Are you sad Christmas is over, and we'll have to
take the sparkle down?

BEN: No dear, my cold hasn't gone yet (manly cough).

ME: And there was me, saying you won't catch colds, now

that you're not working in an office full of women who are often getting colds – their naughty little cold germs jumping onto you – then you come home and they hurl themselves onto me, expecting me to welcome them with open nostrils......... When you went for your wintry walk on the beach over Christmas with Bill, I told you to wrap-up warm, but did you listen to me?

BEN:        No dear.

* * * * * * * *

7.31 p.m.

We sit, silently sipping and gazing into the fire – watching delicate yellow flames licking chunky brown logs. We crunch on cheese and onion crisps, lusciously licking our salty lips and smiling at the serene scene – warming and golden as the whisky behind the bar. While freezing cold rain lashes and crashes against the window panes, thunder rumbles in the heavens, and lightning flashes like Christmas tree lights about to expire.

ME:         Did you know, the golden flower of St John's Wort was worn on St John's Eve because it was supposed to ward off thunderbolts and evil spirits?

BEN:        That's interesting...... *crunch..... crunch.*

ME:         We should get one of those imitation log burners, it will make the sitting room cosier, and they make you feel warm, even when the heat isn't turned on – the logs glow such wonderful orangey-reds and golds. And there's leaping flames with little sparks!

BEN: Leaping flames and sparks eh! Sounds magical.......
*crunch...... crunch...... crunch.*

ME: For now I think I'll keep the cards and decorations up – they make the room nice and cosy. Especially the gold tinsel.

BEN: Anything you say dear..... *munch..... munch.*

ME: And I'd like to keep the cards up in the kitchen too. Did you notice how arty I've been with the cards; red, green and white designs to match our red and white tulips and their green leaves. The curve of the Santa's red coat echoing the curve of the red tulips. The curves of the Christmas tree branches, matching the curves of the tulip leaves – the bendy stems echoing the curves of leaping red and green reindeer?

BEN: The snowy hills match the curves of the white tulips.

ME: You noticed!

BEN: Just guessing. Shall I get green and red peppers and a fresh white cauli to sit with your creation, so you can take arty photos?

ME: That sounds fun. I'll leave the jolly Santa and Rudolph dangling from the cupboard doors too.

BEN: OK...... *sip..... sip.*

*He was far more cheerful*
*Now that he was beerful*
*And no longer tearful*

ME: It's true. Couples who live together for a long time

*do* become alike!

\* \* \* \* \* \* \* \*

ME: Ooh, it's so lovely to be out and having a relaxing time, instead of enduring an appointment at the dentist, doctor, test for cancer, optician or –

BEN: A visit to your family.

ME: I didn't say that (smiling).

BEN: I could *hear* you not saying it. You'd still be recovering from a family visit, and be too fatigued to leave the house today if you'd seen them at Christmas.

ME: True.

BEN: Pity they all had colds and flu.

ME: Yes. A great pity...... *sip*...... *sip*...... I noticed there wasn't the usual sound of constant police sirens from town on Christmas day. Families were too full of festive food and flopped in front of the TV, to fight with each other.

BEN: Yeah.

ME: It *is a pity* the nice young tenants next door with little Dottie, had to move away so soon to live with the in-laws. I was just getting used to them, and their Christmas card was so sweet, with wildlife sitting around a sparkly tree, *and* I thought we'd finally got some good neighbours after *all* these years. Let's hope the next ones are just as pleasant.

BEN:    Yep. Fancy another bag of crisps?

ME:    Why not! Let's go mad and have a different flavour. Indulge ourselves. I still feel Christmassy....... Did you know otters can eat a quarter of their weight in food every day, not just at Christmas?

BEN:    Wonderful.

ME:    I expect you'd like to be Golden Wonder *full*.

BEN:    Yes dear.

* * * * * * * *

ME:    There's a young couple in the corner, fighting quietly (moving eyes to the left). She looks like she's about to throw her Prosecco in his sulky face. Maybe she caught him kissing her best mate under the mistletoe!

BEN:    Oh yeah. And he looks like he wants to throw brandy over her brassy blonde head, and set light to her hair, like a Christmas pudding.

ME:    Shame. This is such a peaceful pub. And it's not long past the season of good will to all men.

BEN:    And women.

ME:    They should be lit-up with love like a Christmas tree, and listening to Phil Collins crooning in the background.

> *Wouldn't you agree*
> *Baby you and me*
> *We've got a groovy kinda' love*

*Groovy kinda' love*
*We've got a groovy kinda' love*

\* \* \* \* \* \* \* \*

7.39 p.m.   At a table nearby, two middle-aged ladies looked a little dismayed. They didn't receive the meal they ordered, and we *couldn't* resist listening to their conversation with the waitress and chef, because I'm a nosey person now, and so is Ben because couples who live together for a long time *do* become alike.

Ladies:   Ooh, excuse me, but I don't think this is what we ordered.

Waitress:   Oh dear, I'm so sorry, what was it you asked for?

Ladies:   Well it's no bother really, we both actually like this, but we didn't want to tuck into it in case it was meant for someone else you see.

Waitress:   I'll just check with the chef, one moment.

Chef:   I'm so sorry! I misread what was on the order, I need new glasses! Let me take that away and I'll get you what you ordered.

Ladies:   Oh no, really, it's no bother and we wouldn't want it to go to waste would we.

Waitress:   But you didn't ask for those did you, really I'm *sooo* sorry. Poor chef, I do scribble things down rather, when we're busy (sounding a little upset now).

Ladies:   Oh no dear, really, don't worry, we don't know how you cope sometimes in your job, we couldn't do it! Please, it's all fine and looks lovely chef, we are fine with it, *honestly!*

Waitress: Well if you're really sure?

Chef: Yes, no problem to change.

Ladies: No that's fine and it looks and smells delicious!

7.45 p.m.
More apologies all round and everyone was happy.

## Tuesday 8th

ME: Did you know pub signs date from the days of mass illiteracy, when customers relied on a picture to convey the name?

BEN: Nope.

ME: Next time we're out and pass old pubs with pictures on their signs, I'll imagine I'm back in the olden days when many people just signed their name with a shaky cross.

BEN: That'll be fun dear, there's plenty of them in our part of the country!

ME: People who sign their names with a shaky cross, or pubs? (giggling)....... I drank in the oldest pub in England once, in my lunch hour when I was at college in Rochester. I can't recall the name, but know it was close to the castle. It was small, and there was supposed to be a monk buried in the wall.

BEN:   I expect you'd like to drink there after hours, when everyone has gone home and talk to the ghost of the monk.

ME:    Sounds good! These very old pubs are often full of spirits.

BEN:   What are you like.

ME:    I encountered the spirit of a monk once, when we stayed at that old place in Lavenham, dating back to the fourteenth century I think, where monks used to live. Remember? With the ornate four-poster beds?

BEN:   Yeah.

ME:    We were about to go out to dinner, and I was standing at the dressing table mirror, wondering if I looked OK, and he just drifted out of the lovely old stone fireplace and smiled at me, as if to say, you look fine dear. It was really nice..... Oh (smiling), I remember your four-poster bed was Jacobean, dark carved wood. It looked creepy, and I couldn't resist lying on the bedcovers, staring up at the canopy, and wondering how many people had died, lying in the bed, looking up at the spooky carvings in the woodwork. Then I started to feel ill and dead creepy and nearly –

BEN:   Scared yourself to death?

* * * * * * * *

ME:    The two ladies who didn't get the meal they ordered in the pub last night were sweet weren't they.

BEN: Yeah. Very English and polite.

ME: Must have been nice for the hard working chef and waitress, who have to deal with complaints.

BEN: Yeah.

ME: And it's great to know the pub does lots of vegetarian and vegan meals now, instead of *only two*, not very tasty sounding vegetarian meals at the end of the menu, to keep the hippies happy. I'd love to celebrate my birthday there. Could you see if their menu is on the internet, so I can enjoy a mouth-watering peruse?

BEN: Certainly dear.

\* \* \* \* \* \* \* \* \*

ME: Ooh, the Moroccan-inspired cauliflower tart in a kale and thyme pastry case sounds tasty. With a baby spinach and leek base, topped with seeds and herb dressing, and served with a slow-roasted tomato sauce. What do you fancy?

BEN: All of them!..... The spiced coconut curry with miso sesame aubergine, broccoli, scorched red chilli and jasmine rice sounds good. And the slow-roasted tomato and almond bake.

ME: Mmm.... Topped with beetroot, carrot, spinach and celeriac. The Mezze flatbread with a creamy hummus base, topped with roasted chick peas, Greek-style salad, seeds, avocado and rocket, and served with salad, sounds very YOU.

BEN: The wholefood salad with leaves, roasted veg, broccoli, avocado, seeds and ginger, lemongrass and pineapple dressing, sounds very YOU.

ME: The pan-fried oyster mushrooms don't appeal to me as a starter, though the dip sounds nice.

BEN: But you love mushrooms?

ME: It's the word oyster. Remember the Oyster House we viewed in Pevensey Bay?

BEN: Yeah.

ME: So dirty and depressing and ugh –

BEN: We could share a baked Camembert with rustic toast, and a spiced fruit and sloe gin chutney.

ME: That would be romantic dear....... The desserts look even more delicious!....... Apple, plum and damson crumble, served with –

BEN: I can't peruse anymore, getting *very hungry* now.

ME: I'm not surprised! You haven't eaten much today, just bananas. I know you're on a diet, but you mustn't crash diet, it's not good for you.

BEN: I'm trying to be super-good after all the Christmas, new year and getting-over-a-cold indulgence.

ME: There's a programme on tonight you should watch, *The Big Fat Lies About Diet And Exercise.* It's about the potential pitfalls of trying to lead a more healthy lifestyle – from the dangers of crash dieting to the unexpected side effects of doing too much exercise. The programme features contributions from nutritionists, dieticians, GPs and fitness trainers, who explain the health benefits of fat and carbohydrates, the addictive quality of sugar, the hazards of diet pills, and what can happen to someone if they eat too many bananas.

BEN:  Thank you dear.

ME:  I wonder what happens when you eat too many bananas.

BEN:  You become more *a-peeling?* (peeling a banana).

ME:  Maybe. I think you could start to turn pale green – say, on a Tuesday. Then by Thursday you'd be a greeny-yellow, and by Sunday –

BEN:  Banana yellow?

ME:  Yes. And the following Tuesday, dark brown freckles begin to appear over the bridge –

BEN:  Of the River Medway?

ME:  Of your nose. Then next day you –

BEN:  Call the doctor?

ME:  Probably. Because the freckles will be bigger and browner and blotchier, *and* have spread down your neck, to your chest, and along your arms, all the way to your black-nailed fingertips. Then by Thursday, the blotchy-brown freckles will have started to join up together and you start to panic because –

BEN:      The doctor doesn't know what's wrong.

ME:      Because by the Sunday your *whole body* will be dark brown blotches and big brown spots. And by the following Saturday there will be barely any yellow patches visible on your skin..... By the end of the week, you're very weak and floppy, and your skin has turned such a dark brown, it looks black. And you end up in hospital, where during the night, while you sleep, a fungus starts to appear in your armpits and your arms drop off, then the same fungus grows at the tops of your legs, and your legs drop off. And the hospital is so understaffed no-one notices. And eventually your head drops off!... Does the thought of eating too many bananas sound less a-*peeling* now?

BEN:      No, not really (munch, munch).

ME:      I went strawberry picking with my family when I was twelve or thirteen. I ate lots of strawberries, turned a bit pink, and little red spots appeared all over my body – I was turning into a strawberry! It was a bit scary. Mum took me to the doctor and I think it was an allergy.... Did you know that eating carrots and red peppers every day gives your skin a healthy glow?

BEN:      Fascinating – have you been drinking my real coffee again? You're a bit buzzy.

ME:      I may have had just one. Or two. Am I a buzzy bee, growing black and yellow stripy fur and sprouting wings. Actually that sounds quite nice. And it must be cool to have five eyes, little antennae, and get to sniff flowers all day.

BEN:     Five eyes?

ME:      Yes. Three simple eyes and two compound eyes.

BEN:     Bees must spend a small fortune at the bee optician.

ME:      They collect Nectar points from Sainsbury's to help with the cost.

BEN:     What are you like.

ME:      I'm a buzzy body in the kitchen, about to prepare a lovely low calorie, nutritious musician's dinner.

BEN:     Musician's dinner? *Beat*-root salad?

ME:      It's a *melody* instead of a *medley* of fresh vegetables, with veggie sausages and *note*-worthy gravy.

BEN:     Music to my ears. Will you cook it on our *stave?*

* * * * * * * *

ME:      You noticed my arty green and white display of Christmas cards and flowers in the kitchen, didn't you.

BEN:     Yes dear.

ME:      Did you note how the tiny gypsophila flower heads were *so like* the snowflakes in the snowy scene. And the red Santa hats on the cartoon cats card were echoed in the curves of the red tulips.

BEN:     Thank you for the wonderful lesson in art appreciation – I'll make the most of it next time I'm in the kitchen.

## Wednesday 9th

2.00 p.m.

BEN:     I see you're about to make a start on your painting by numbers.

ME:      I am at last! I'm finally getting a *round-tuit*.

BEN:     They *can* be hard to find.

ME:      It's going to be a HUGE challenge because it's as big as a thousand piece jigsaw puzzle.

BEN:     Instead of picking up hundreds of little jigsaw puzzle pieces you'll be –

ME:      Painstakingly painting, over a thousand little colourful, curly, swirly, blobby shapes with numbers in the middle, telling me what colours I should use to create a beautiful technicolour portrait of a cat.

BEN:     What sort of cat is it?!

ME:      A spooky looking feline – like a psychedelic statue of an Egyptian cat. You get a breed of cat called a Parisian.... no..... Peruvian..... Pomeranian..... that's a wee dog..... Persian....... Persian Blue!........ Maybe the cat is an Egyptian red, yellow, green and Prussian Blue!

BEN:     Of course, why didn't I think of that.

ME:      It's about twenty-five times bigger than the little completed picture they give you so it'll be –

BEN:     Twenty-five times spookier.

ME:      And more striking. *I love it!*

BEN:     It'll keep you quiet – I mean occupied for weeks.

ME:      Months probably, by the look of it.

BEN:     Even better – I mean that'll be nice for you.

ME:      It will. I imagine I'll do a little most days. Maybe an hour or two with rests, on a good day.

BEN:     Two minutes, on a not-so-good day.

ME:      It'll be like climbing a hill in the countryside – Derbyshire or Yorkshire. And resting, sitting on the grass when I start to tire, knowing that the effort will be worth it when I finally reach the top.

BEN:     And enjoy the view.

ME:      Yes, a wonderful patchwork of greens, of the countryside.

BEN:     In this case, a patchwork of multi-coloured cat.

ME:      There *are* lots of colours. Seventeen delightful little pots of acrylic paint. *Four* shades of green and blue – look! Number thirteen is a gorgeous Prussian blue.

BEN:     You went off that colour when you attempted a five hundred piece jigsaw puzzle, a few years ago – a painting by Waterhouse, with a *lot* of Prussian blue.

ME:     Oh yes, I'd forgotten about that. Looks like there's not much of it in the painting, phew! Number nine is a pretty turquoise, and number twelve is one of my favourite blues – cobalt. Nice isn't it.

BEN:    Yeah, very nice.

ME:     This one is a *beautiful* deep purple. It's number one. And number two – isn't this a lovely lilac!...... The greens are *great!* Number eleven is lime green and number eight is olive –

BEN:    I get the picture dear.

ME:     No. *Noo.* You won't get the picture for weeks. Not until I've completed the painting. I think I'll start with the bright red, because it's an energy giving colour. Although turquoise and lime green are too.

BEN:    Decisions, decisions.

ME:     I'd like to start with the heart on the cat's forehead. That's the red, so decision made. My achievement for the day!

BEN:    Well done, I'm sure you'll put your *heart* into it.

ME:     Very amusing (big smile). I'm not sure if I'll paint all the red bits first, there's so many! How many do you think there are? Have a guess. Look at the tiny finished version.

BEN:    Twenty?

ME:        There's about *sixty!* My eyes went a bit cross-eyed, trying to count. Guess how many are turquoise.

BEN:       Must I?

ME:        Have a go, I won't ask again!

BEN:       Twenty-five?

ME:        Close, about thirty. And there's over fifty lime green bits.

BEN:       Have you counted them all?!

ME:        No, that's all. I was just bored. And curious.

BEN:       Looking at all the detail I can see why it's going to take so long to paint.

ME:        I'm looking forward to it. Every time I get bored of a colour, I'll change to another one.

BEN:       As you climb your hill in Yorkshire or Derbyshire, you'll change the colour of your boots every ten minutes. But you'll need someone to carry them for you.

ME:        Yes, you!

\* \* \* \* \* \* \* \*

5.30 p.m.

BEN:       Why the long face?

ME:        I was really looking forward to *Coronation Street* tonight. It was *so good* on Monday – Gemma lost her temper in the Rovers, Gina was trapped in the office, and Liz realised it was Jenny who knocked her down with her car in the street, not Jonny.

BEN: Sorry I missed that.

ME: But I can't watch it tonight. TV Weekly says Tim takes a call from the prison to say something awful has happened to Sally.

BEN: Never mind, I'm sure things will get better soon. Is there something else you can look forward to watching?

ME: Oh yes! I've just seen, Phil and Kirstie are on later.

BEN: Phil and Kirstie?

ME: Phil Spencer and Kirstie Allsopp. They present that property advice series, *Kirstie and Phil's Love It Or List It*. And *Location, Location, Location*.

BEN: I've heard of the last one.

ME: They were in our town last year, doing that programme. Almost as exciting as when Peter Andre was in our town!

BEN: I'm sure it was.

ME: At the end, they meet a couple in a pub, in the town they are in, to ask what property they'd like to buy. Then Phil or Kirstie ring the vendors, to suggest an offer the couple would like to put in – it's really good, has me on the edge of my seat with anticipation!

BEN:    I'm sure it does.

ME:    Guess which pub they went to?

BEN:    No idea.

ME:    Have a guess.

BEN:    Must I?

ME:    It'll be fun.

BEN:    Will it?

ME:    I'll give you a clue. It's one we've been to over the years.

BEN:    The Pilot?..... Walnut Tree?

ME:    No.

BEN:    First and Last?..... The White Horse?

ME:    Close. To do with horses.

BEN:    The Horseshoes?

ME:    *YES!*..... The one we went to yesterday!

BEN:    But it's not in Maidstone.

ME:    Oh, *true*. Not far outside though. And I can see why they chose that one – we did! I expect they wanted a posh country pub with lots of lovely log fires, and plenty of room for a camera crew and entourage. They sat not far from where we sat.

BEN: And you wish you'd been there, to give them a little wave?

ME: I do. By the sounds in the background, the pub was fairly busy.

BEN: Never mind dear. Next time we go, we could sit in the seats that they sat in.

ME: Kirstie doesn't do just property programmes, she's very arty and crafty too! I watched her in *Kirstie's Hand Made Christmas* last month. Now she's doing *Kirstie Fills Your House For Free,* and the other one.... *Kirstie's Pleasures.....* no, *Kirstie's Prezzies....* *Kirstie's Treasures......* no.

BEN: *Kirstie's Treasure Island?*

ME: *Kirstie's Handmade Prezzies.......* no.

BEN: *Kirstie's Handmade Treasures* (perusing TV Weekly).

ME: Yes!

BEN: So glad we've got that sorted dear.

\* \* \* \* \* \* \* \*

ME: Did you notice there's a programme on tonight, *How To Lose Weight Well?* Caroline and Charmaine have a week to slim down for a spa day and try the cabbage soup and potato diet. David and John go on six-week plans to lose weight for a friend's wedding, while Karen and Tracey take a stab at the metabolic diet and genetic diet, in a bid to get in shape for a summer holiday.

BEN: Sounds fascinating.

ME: I read in Celebrity Weekly that Robbie Williams is the new face of Weight Watchers.

BEN: I'm sure he's thrilled.

ME: There's a photo of Robbie with his family on a winter break, on a beach somewhere exotic – he looks very slim and fit.

BEN: Lucky him.

ME: There's another programme on tonight that should be really good, *Death on the Tyne*.

BEN: Why, have you seen it?

ME: No, but it's the comedy sequel to *Murder on the Blackpool Express,* which was dead funny.

BEN: Oh yeah, did you nearly *die* laughing?

ME: I did!.......... I've just read, *Death on the Tyne* is a series of murders that take place after an *overweight curry*. I must have my M.E. eyeballs in today.

BEN: What should you have read?

ME: The murders take place on an *overnight ferry*.

BEN: Your version sounds better.

ME: Thanks.

BEN: I could *murder* a curry!

## Thursday 10th

10.00 am

ME:       It was so lovely out there (pointing to building site) when it snowed, and there was no-one around. So peaceful. All was calm.

BEN:     All was bright.

ME:       *Silent night*
*Holy night*
*All was calm*
*All was bright*

*At the moment*
*The weather is mild*
*Though it's gonna turn*
*Windy and wild*

*I long for heavenly peace*
*Snowy white heavenly peace*

BEN:     Wishing for snow again dear?

ME:       Yes, but at least it's not too noisy on the site at the moment – just a bit of work going on at the far end, removing rubble. The houses in our street are enjoying a rest from trembling all day.

BEN:     I'll put a new battery in your snowmen snow globe, then you can sit it in the window –

ME:       And pretend it's snowing (big sigh, head on one side).

11.30 a.m.  The weatherman said it was going to turn very windy, but it's already getting extremely gusty-with-the-promise-of-gales. The green flags around the building site, advertising the wonderful-housing-development-to-be are fluttering *so madly,* I wouldn't be surprised if they were soon in shreds.

11.31 a.m.  I watch two crows, huge black wings flapping, swoop over a JCB. Two seagulls glide, circling over the chip shop opposite the far end of the site. Two workmen plod over a mound of earth, shouting and flapping their arms at each other.

11.32 a.m.  I wish for peace on earth and goodwill to all men.

12.42 p.m.  The leaves on the trees at the end of our garden flutter like hands of little children saying goodbye to granny and grandad.

12.43 p.m.  Three collared doves peck at peanuts on the bird table. Then there's a lot of flapping of grey wings when a squirrel appears, bounding along the fence towards them.

1.50 p.m.  There's more flapping on *60 Minute Makeover,* as Linda Barker flies into designer's-last-minute-panic – a makeover for Maisy is almost over but there's still *so much to do!*....... Candles and glass jars to be artily placed on a shelf...... a table laid stylishly with shiny cutlery and fresh, lime green napkins... straightening of pictures on the walls...... a flower arrangement to be rearranged.... bright red cushions carefully placed at angles on a black sofa.

1.55 p.m.  Linda has calmed down, now the makeover is over. And I feel peaceful, just sitting, watching my snow globe – snowflakes softly swirling around snowmen who are smiling at me, wearing red and green stripey scarves and black top hats. I smile back.

2.00 p.m.  Feel in a creative mood – time for a little painting by numbers. More bright red and green I think. Which green?..... Lime green, like the napkins in *60 Minute Makeover* or a dark green, like one of the stripey scarves worn by a snowman?..... *Both!*

* * * * * * * *

5.10 p.m.

BEN:  What's making you giggle?

ME:  I've got my M.E. eyeballs in again. Just read in TV Weekly, there's a programme about a man who waves his tail when he meets his wife.

BEN:  What should you have read?

ME:  A man *weaves a tale* about how he met his wife.

BEN:  I expect if men had tails, they would wag them if they saw a female they fancied.

ME:  Did your tail wag when you met me?

BEN:  Of course dear.

ME:  I also read in TV Weekly that Alan Carr chats to Kylie Minogue tonight about her career and surprises her with flowers.

BEN:  That sounds OK.

ME:      I should have read, that the programme was made to surprise her *followers*.

BEN:     He might surprise her with flowers!

ME:      I'd like to watch the show to see if he does, but *Grand Designs* is on at the same time.

\* \* \* \* \* \* \* \* \*

5.45 p.m.

BEN:     What's making you cackle now?

ME:      Look at the label on this can of lentil and vegetable soup. I thought it had a warning on the front, a heart warning. And that it was thickened with rough-chopped root vegetables and split ends!

BEN:     Ah, it's *hearty and warming,* thickened with rough-chopped vegetables and *split lentils*. Is painting by numbers making your eyes extra tired?

ME:      I must admit it's more tiring than I thought it would be. I'd forgotten just how much concentration it takes to paint, and I didn't think I'd become fatigued so quickly. BUT it does make time fly and I'll get there in the end.

BEN:     In the split end?

ME:      Yes dear. It'll feel like a HUGE achievement.

BEN:     That's good.

ME:      And I do enjoy stroking thick liquid onto canvas –

feels sort of therapeutic.

BEN:      Or what you call *very-peutic*.

ME:      Or Verity-peutic!

BEN:      Is it like stroking Diamanda's soft, silky fur?

ME:      *It is!* But it's easy to get carried away, forget to rest, and though you feel fatigue coming on, you're enjoying yourself and thinking – I'll just paint one more bit then I'll stop – then you do just one more bit, and then you do another, then another, then –

BEN:      I get the picture.

ME:      No, *noo*. You won't get the picture until it's finally completed. One day!

BEN:      You must pace yourself or you'll end up so fatigued, you'll not be able to paint for days.

ME:      You're right. And I have to remember how –

BEN:      Many women it takes to change a light bulb?

ME:      I know you are going to tell me.

BEN:      One. She just holds it in place while the world revolves around her.

ME:      Very amusing dear. I was going to say, I have to remember *how long* it takes for paint to dry. When you are colouring in with felt-tip pens, it only takes seconds. When painting, I have found myself resting my hand on a not-quite-dried-yet bit, and smudging my hard work. And I have to remember when I'm taking a break, to sit the canvas upright, and how –

BEN: Many psychiatrists it takes to change a light bulb?

ME: Enlighten me.

BEN: Only one. But the bulb has to *really* want to change.

ME: Ha, ha, ha! – What was I saying?...... Oh, yes. I have to remember how it's *so easy* to forget to sit the canvas upright when you suddenly feel *ever so* tired.

BEN: So mischievous little furry paws don't tread on it?

ME: Yes. Diamanda nearly got bright red paw pads, like the soles of designer shoes.

BEN: She'd be a puss with posh paws.

ME: Little Miss Diamanda de Signer Paws.

## Friday 11th

10.00 a.m. It's still a windy world outside. A wild and windy, green flag-flapping day around the building site.

10.05 a.m. Winter weary workmen, wearing yellow waistcoats, continue to flap their arms at each other.

10.06 a.m. There are no big black crows in sight on the site.

10.07 a.m. I feel some verse coming on.

*Workmen on the building site*

*There is not a crow in flight*

10.20 a.m.  Sipping a refreshing minty tea – do I feel more verse coming on?

10.21 a.m.  No. Not today.

11.05 a.m.  Ben sends me a text message from town:

> I SIMPLY DON'T BELIEVE IT – AFTER GOING TO SERIOUS LENGTHS TO PACK LAPTOP SECURELY FOR RETURN AND REPAIR – THE NICE ARGOS LADY LOOKED IT ALL UP AND THEY DON'T OFFER REPAIRS ON THAT MODEL, JUST A REFUND AND REPLACEMENT – FEELIN EXTREMELY MELDREW

11.06 a.m.  I smile as I recall Victor Meldrew, who is always in an angry flap, saying he *simply doesn't believe it,* in *One foot In The Grave.* Then before I have time to send a sympathetic reply, he sends another text message:

> HAVIN CAPPUCCINO TO CALM DOWN

11.07 a.m.  I'm tempted to reply, telling him about a similar scenario I'd seen recently on a TV reality show, which was far worse than his experience, and very costly for the young man, so he should think himself lucky. But this was not the time. So I replied:

> SORRY TO HEAR THAT – NEVER MIND – THE EXERCISE WILL DO YOU GOOD X

11.25 a.m.  I'm watching *Say Yes to the Dress.* Samantha is in a fearful flap. She has put on far too much weight, and is unable to fit into the mermaid style wedding dress with a sweetheart neckline. She simply *cannot fit* into the fit & flare satin dress covered in beautiful, sparkly bling. Or the super Cinderella dress – a timeless classic with layers of organza. Her face is a veil of tears.

1.10 p.m.    Rachel is in a panicky flap in *Friends*. She is about to meet her very controlling father for dinner, and is going to tell him she is pregnant. And she knows he will *demand* to know who the father is, and *when* is he going to marry her? And when she tells him she's not going to get married, he will demand to know *WHY NOT?* At least she won't have to worry about squeezing into a wedding dress.

2.00 p.m.    I'm feeling very *un-flapped*. Ever so calm, peaceful and creative – think I will do more painting by numbers. No squeezing of paint tubes, just dipping of paintbrush into delightful little pots of rainbow colours. Which colour shall I begin with today?

2.01 p.m.    Red? Yellow? Green? Blue?

2.02 p.m.    Purple, I think......... Yes, purple.

* * * * * * * *

4.25 p.m.

ME:    It's a pity you couldn't get your laptop repaired after all the effort you went to, parcelling it up. But you are most fortunate that you're not the young man I saw on a TV reality show recently. He lived in America, and wanted to send an enormous plasma TV to his mother and sister in Brazil. The place he took it to, parcelled it up really well, and when he was told the price of the postage, his face was a picture. I think it was going to cost a thousand dollars! This was far too expensive. But he still had to pay for the packaging, and was stuck with a TV he didn't want, so I think he was a lot more cheesed-off than you!

BEN:     Thank you dear, that makes me feel a whole lot better. How's the painting of the spooky cat coming along?

ME:      Much better now that I'm taking more rests and not smudging the paint before it dries. I used purple today – look!

BEN:     Very nice.

ME:      It looks good next to the turquoise and lime green. And doesn't the red look *RADIANT* next to the lime green! The green makes the red look *very red* –

BEN:     Verity Red!

ME:      And the red makes the green, *very green.*

BEN:     Splendid.

ME:      Oh, and look at the lilac next to the turquoise – so pretty.

BEN:     Truly magnificent.

ME:      The greens in the eyes are going to stand out beautifully, and *glow* when surrounded by the black. They will look hypnotic and magical. The colours in the whole portrait will be jewel-like when I've painted the black background. And –

BEN: I get the picture.

ME: No, *noo*. You won't get the picture until I've finished it!

BEN: Of course dear.

\* \* \* \* \* \* \* \*

*Painting is silent poetry, and poetry is painting that speaks.*

Simonides

# February

8.43 a.m.

BEN:     Looking good.... Beautiful eyes!

ME:      Thank you – I take it you mean the eyes in my cat painting, not me.

BEN:     Yeah.

ME:      For a moment I was transported back, years ago, when we first met.

BEN:     You still have nice eyes dear.

ME:      Thanks – when I can keep them open. Can't stop yawning today. Kept waking up in the night after some weird dreams. Well, more weird than I've had for a long time. I was working on my painting, when the cat very slowly took on the features of the Mona Lisa. Her enigmatic smile turned into a grin with cat fangs, then her mouth opened *really wide* and she cackled in a *most evil* way.

BEN:     Not a nice little cackle like yours.

ME:      No, it was quite frightening. Then the canvas turned black, and the room turned pitch dark, and I was trapped in the toilet at the clinic in London again, sitting on the cold floor. I called out to you but no sound came out of my mouth. Then luminous spiders appeared. They were all the colours in my painting and crawled *all over* the walls and floor, and my flesh is creeping, just recalling when they started to crawl over me. Still feel a bit shaky.

BEN: I'll get you a camomile tea dear, and I have a joke for you. A man goes to the doctor and says he can't sleep. What does the doctor reply?

ME: No idea (yawning like a cat).

BEN: Sit on the edge of the bed and you'll soon drop off.

ME: That's a good one (cackling nicely).

\* \* \* \* \* \* \* \*

BEN: Got another joke for you. Guess who I bumped into in Specsavers?

ME: No idea. Who did you bump into?

BEN: Guess who I... *bumped* into in... *Specsavers?*

ME: Oh! (nice loud cackle).

BEN: The eyes in your painting *do* seem to follow me around the room, like the Mona Lisa.

ME: Or a cat, with a *give-me-a-tuna-treat-or-else* stare.

BEN: Yeah – I've just been meowed at *meaningfully.*

ME: You'll be having nightmares next – the Mona Lisa following you around the house, meowing at you, demanding tuna. Or when you are awake, seeing the whiskers twitch in the painting and the eyes blink – the multicolours playing tricks with your brain.

BEN: Diamanda was sitting and staring at it yesterday, with menacing eyes and tail twitching.

ME: Maybe she's communicating with the spirit of the cat that inspired the painting. Or she's been having cat nightmares too. I heard her growling in her sleep the other day, and her paws were doing little clawing movements.

BEN: Maybe she's dreaming of using the canvas as a scratching post.

ME: I'd better keep it out of naughty paws reach.

BEN: Good idea.

ME: Sometimes, when I look at the small print of what the painting will look like when it's finished, I imagine the cat is thinking – *IS THIS REALLY HAPPENING?* Because it was a black cat, that accidentally drank a witch's potion that brings more colour into your life, and its coat turned multicolours.

BEN: A technicolour cat's dreamcoat!

ME: Yes (cackling nicely again).Think I'll bring the nose alive next – paint black around the red and lilac tip, then mustard, apple green and red on the bridge of the nose. I know I'll start to crave mustard when I open the little number fifteen pot of paint, it's so *mustardy*.

BEN: Better put mustard on the shopping list then! And a choc pot for when you open the little..... Where is it?.... Ah.... Here it is, number four pot of chocolate coloured paint.

ME:     I fancy a KitKat now, any left in the cupboard?

BEN:    One.

ME:     Oh goody, I'll pop it in the fridge so it goes *nice'n' cold'n'crispy* – I need perking up, so I can continue with my masterpiece. I'll hide it under some veg –

BEN:    The painting? It won't fit in the fridge!

ME:     Very funny. I don't want you to be tempted to have a chocolatey treat and spoil your diet.

BEN:    That's thoughtful of you dear.

ME:     Look at this pot (opening pot number seven), it's a lovely apple green. It'll make you want to munch a nice, fresh, crispy apple.

BEN:    Not working I'm afraid, and the number fourteen –

ME:     Ah, toffee brown. Makes you fancy toffee, me too. Whatever you do, don't look at the gift catalogue that arrived yesterday – my mouth *actually watered* when I looked at all hazelnut, raspberry and pink champagne truffles, tins of clotted cream short-bread, rich chocolate cookies, and all-butter biscuits. Fudge, caramels and –

BEN:    Hang on (plodding to kitchen, returning with KitKat, opening little red and white packet, then breaking off two chocolaty fingers). One for you, one for me.

ME:     Thanks (giggling).

10.44 a.m.  I'm in the kitchen, sipping de-caf coffee, enjoying a crispy finger of KitKat, and watching two collared doves (their plumage, the softest, loveliest grey) enjoying a nutty treat.

10.45 a.m.  The garden is starting to look like a Victoria sponge cake (with wildlife cake decorations), lightly sprinkled with icing sugar.

10.46 a.m.  Inspired by chocolate and the sweet scene before my eyes, I softly sing to myself.

*Oh the weather outside is frightful*
*But the fire is so delightful*
*And since we've no place to go*

*Let it snow!*
*Let it snow!*
*Let it snow!*

10.47 a.m.  Since I've no place to go, I wish for snow. But not too much. Ben will be off out soon and away for the night, and if we have lots of snow he may be unable to return home for days.

10.48 a.m.  My coffee, usually black, tastes so nice with sweetened soya milk, I feel inspired to sing once more.

*Oh the weather outside is frightful*
*But the fire is so delightful*
*And since I've no place to go*

*Sweet and low!*
*Sweet and low!*
*Sweet and low!*

\* \* \* \* \* \* \* \*

11.06 a.m.     The house is too quiet now that Ben has driven off to visit his sister Julia and her husband Paul, who live in a lovely village near Colchester. It's the first time in years I've wished for *just a little* snowfall.

11.31 a.m.     I'm perched on the bed, home alone (apart from a purring Diamanda in the window), staring out of the window. The building site is not a pretty site, but is improved with a sprinkling of snow. Three huge piles of rubble and earth, bring to mind pyramid-shaped piles of chocolate cake crumbs, dusted generously with desiccated coconut.

11.32 a.m.     I want to sneak into the building site with three big shiny, red beach balls and place a ball on top of each mound.

11.33 a.m.     I do like a cake decorated with a shiny, red glacé cherry, or a white cupcake with a cherry on top.

11.45 a.m.     Staring in bathroom mirror. Not a pretty sight. But could be improved with a touch of sparkly, pink blusher and lippy, and maybe a cherry red beret perched on my head.

11.50 a.m.     Today's post arrived, and after putting the boring looking envelopes to one side, I settled down to enjoy a leisurely peruse of the more colourful post – Joe Browns catalogue and ALDI, who were advertising their special buys for Valentine's Day.

11.51 a.m.     The scented candles looked and sounded nice, especially the soft pink one, scented with a blend of roses, violets and vanilla. The cookies with a heart-shaped raspberry filling looked *most delicious*, so did the fresh, juicy looking strawberries dipped in plain chocolate with Amaretto.

11.52 a.m.     Must make a Valentine's Day card for Ben. Hope I'll get a tasty treat on the day. Maybe I'll just happen to leave ALDI's special buys on the coffee table, instead of throwing it into the recycling bin.

11.56 a.m.     Joe Browns is full of deliciously pretty, fruity fashions – the vintage dress with oranges and lemons design, pineapple print gypsy top, and the capri pants (black with strawberries and strawberry leaf design) catch my eye.

12.07 p.m.     As I munch a sweet snack of banana on wholemeal toast, sprinkled with grated plain chocolate, I enjoy a sweet daydream – I'm reclining on a raspberry red velvet chez longue, feeling pretty because my maid has done my hair, nails and make-up, and I'm wearing a vintage dress with oranges and lemons design. Rose and violet scented candles flicker and fill the air with their flowery fragrance, and the mantel-shelf is full of Valentine cards from my man and admirers in the charming, peaceful village where I live. Holding a Jane Austen novel in one hand, and the other hand delicately picking up a fresh, juicy strawberry dipped in plain chocolate with Amaretto, I smile beatifically.

12.10 p.m.     The ringtone on my mobile phone calls me back to reality. Ben has sent a text message:

ARRIVED SAFELY X

12.11 p.m.     I reply:

GREAT – HAVE A GOOD TIME – LOVE TO J AND P XXX

## Saturday 2nd

More snow fell in the night. I had woken up in the wee small hours, after dreaming about pine martens feeding on strawberries dipped in chocolate and barn owls feeding on cherries in the Cairngorms, in Scotland – no doubt inspired by last night's viewing of *Winterwatch* on BBC 2. I had sat, watching the snowflakes fall on a moonlit mound of earth on the building site, looking very much like a pile of chocolate crumbs and crushed nuts, being sprinkled with icing sugar. After a little while, my eyes started to droop and I curled up under the bed covers again, to dream of pine martens and barn owls feeding on chocolate crumbs and crushed nuts sprinkled with icing sugar.

10.07 a.m.   It's starting to rain.

10.08 a.m.   As always, love to just watch the raindrops splashing down the window pane and listen to the tippy-tapping sound, feeling thankful that I'm indoors, in the warm and dry. The mounds of earth on the site now look like stale, plain chocolate cake. And one mound looks like stale, milk chocolate mixed with walnuts – or I should say bits-of-wall nuts.

10.09 a.m.   The site of stale chocolate is not putting me off chocolate. And I'm happy to see more snow on the hills around our valley. Or is it mist?

10.10 a.m.   Distance glasses on. Yes, definitely snow. Lovely.

10.11 a.m.   Woken out of daydream again by my mobile. Text from Ben:

SNOWING HERE – NOT MUCH SO JOURNEY HOME SHUD BE OK – GOIN TO SAINS ON WAY HOME – WANT ANYTHING?

10.12 a.m.  I replied:

PLAIN CHOC PLZ

And felt very pleased with myself for not texting what I *really, really wanted* – coffee and walnut cake, cupcakes with a glacé cherry on top, strawberries dipped in plain chocolate with Amaretto and......

*That* Spice Girls song has popped into my head – Oh God, it'll be in my head all day.

*I'll tell you what I want*
*What I really, really want*
*I'll tell you what I want*
*What I really, really want*

With a little change of lyrics.

*I wanna, I wanna*
*I wanna, I wanna*
*I really, really, really want*
*A slice 'o'cake now*

10.14 a.m.  ALDI's cookies with a heart-shaped raspberry filling would go nicely with a cuppa too – give me an incentive to paint the second coat on the heart in my Mona Lisa cat's forehead (the number 5 is still showing through the first coat). Will resist the urge to text Ben asking him to pop into ALDI.

10.15 a.m.  I stroke Diamanda's little black forehead and she purrs out love. She has a slightly Mona Lisa look about her – the faintest enigmatic smile, and paws crossed, as if to say, *'Paint me instead, I'm far more inspiring than that silly old painting by numbers –*

*What are you thinking? Give me a salmon treat for sitting so still, like the best artist's model in the world, not twitching an ear or a whisker'.*

10.16 a.m.   I gently caress Diamanda's delicate-as-a-rose-petal ear and decide to paint black around the turquoise and green shapes in the cat painting's ears, when I've mended (I mean painted) the red heart. Then maybe I'll doze off to an episode of *Heartbeat*.

\* \* \* \* \* \* \* \*

4.07 p.m.   Ben returned home safe and sound.

BEN:   Ahh (taking off jacket and shoes), nice to be home. I know what you've been up to (stroking Diamanda as she leans against his leg, then flops on his feet).

ME:   Me or Diamanda?

BEN:   You!

ME:   Really? I can assure you it's not much (giggling).

BEN:   You've got black paint on your nose and cheek.

ME:   Ah, yes (peering in sitting room mirror), that's why the postman grinned at me.

BEN:   Got you a surprise. Close your eyes and open your paws.

ME:   Oh, lovely!

BEN:   Both eyes.

ME:        Yes.

BEN:       Don't open yet, have a sniff and see if you can guess
           what the scent is.

ME:        Ooh!......... The fragrance has reached my sensitive
           witchy nose *already*........ deliciously sweet....... and
           a little like....... the smell of a Christmas tree.

BEN:       Open eyes.

ME:        I'd never have guessed. Wild gorse – the smell of
           Cornish lanes in springtime, with vanilla and a hint
           of coconut.

BEN:       I thought they were very YOU.

ME:        Yes, *very me*, thank you! And a gorgeous fern green
           colour. I'll pop one in a tea light holder and sit it
           with my fairies and unicorn. I imagine Cornish fairy
           folk and pixies love the scent of wild gorse.

BEN:       Yes dear, I expect unicorns like to munch on wild
           gorse too.


## Sunday 3rd

10.23 a.m.

ME:        You'll never guess what I've just seen on the bird
           table. It's a bird I've seen occasionally in the country-
           side, but *NEVER* on our bird table.

BEN:       An eagle?

ME:        No dear.

BEN:       Do enlighten me.

ME:        Have another guess.

BEN:       Must I?

ME:        Yes, it'll be fun.

BEN:       A heron?

ME:        No.

BEN:       Hawk?

ME:        No.

BEN:       Owl?

ME:        No.

BEN:       Partridge?

ME:        Have another guess.

BEN:       Woodpecker?

ME:        No.

BEN:       Magpie?

ME:        *Yes!*..... That was fun wasn't it!

BEN:       I'm *truly exhausted* with excitement.

ME: Close up, the magpie is quite a striking bird – the beautiful blue and white feathers seem to glow amongst the black feathers. It strutted about squawking like a crow.

BEN: Magpies *are* a member of the crow family.

ME: I didn't know you knew anything about birds!

BEN: I'm full of surprises dear, though I'm not going to *crow* about it.

10.46 a.m.

BEN: What's that form you're filling in?

ME: A survey for the RSPB – I've been doing a bird-watch for them.

BEN: So, what birds visit us then?

ME: Have a guess.

BEN: Why did I ask (rolling eyes). Must I? I'm still worn out with excitement.

ME: Just have one guess then.

BEN: Robin (yawning).

ME: Correct! We're also visited by blue tits, coal tits, chaffinches, collared doves, wood pigeons, sometimes a jay or a sparrow, blackbirds and a thrush. And of course the usual gang of pigeons every morning.

BEN: Marvellous. I'd better order some more peanuts for madam's menagerie. And you should add magpie to your list.

ME: Oh yes. Thanks.

BEN: I'm off into town in a few minutes, want anything?

ME: Erm.... just thinking.... got birds on the brain.

BEN: You do twitter away sometimes dear, and your hair *does* look a bit like the building of a bird's nest in progress!

ME: Thank you for the compliments.... Ah, condiments! We need ground black pepper and sea salt...... and capsules. I need more evening primrose oil.... Oh, and Celebrity Weekly – I'm in need of some nice juicy, delicious gossip.

BEN: I'd better write a list.

ME: It's OK I'll do it.

BEN: You and your lists!

ME: Do you know what my favourite list to make is?

BEN: Things for me to do?

ME: No, it's things to take when we go away for a weekend. Secondly, I like making Christmas lists for food treats and gifts. But thinking about it, making *round-tuit* lists for you ought to be top of my list.

BEN: Lucky me.

ME:        Here's your list....... When you said I should add
           *magpie* to my bird list, I thought I'd like to see
           *apple pie* on a shopping list.

BEN:       Great, haven't had apple pie for ages.

ME:        And I made another list, you'll never guess what of.

BEN:       I can't wait to hear.

ME:        Well, when I wrote condiments, capsules and Celebri-
           ty Weekly on your list, I thought to myself, there's
           lots of things I enjoy beginning with **C**. So I made a
           list. I'll read it out to you.

           **C**ats
           **C**hocolate
           **C**elebrity Weekly
           **C**loud watching
           **C**ondiments
           **C**oronation Street
           **C**andles
           **C**atalogues
           **C**ornetto

           Not sure I can add capsules to the list. I appreciate
           them, the good they do, but I don't really enjoy
           taking them. Oh, maybe I will add them to the list.

BEN:       Your life must be endless fun.

ME:        Ooh! I've thought of another one! **C**rystals.

BEN:       I'm off now.

ME:        **C**amomile tea!

BEN:        Have you run out?

ME:         No, just adding to my list.

* * * * * * * *

11.05 a.m.  I send Ben a text message:

            CAULIFLOWER

11.10 a.m.  He replied:

            WHICH LIST ARE YOU ADDING THAT TO DEAR?

11.11 a.m.  I cackled (nicely) and replied:

            BOTH - THANX

12.16 p.m.

BEN:        Here you are. Nice fresh cauliflower, condiments, capsules and Celebrity Weekly. Apple pie. And I got cupcakes with a cherry on top because –

ME:         The lady loves a cherry on top! And it's –

BEN:        Another one to add to the list! I thought you'd like some flowers too.

ME:         Lovely!..... **C**hrysanthemums? **C**arnations?

BEN:        No (laughing) but you'll love the *colours*. Close your eyes.

ME:         OK.

BEN:     Open now.

ME:     Oh, gorgeous scent!

BEN:     *And* you have scented candles.

ME:     With the fragrance of Cornish lanes in the springtime. Cornwall! I've loved all my holidays there – that must go on my list.

BEN:     I expect you like Devonshire *cream* teas too.

ME:     That's five more words. What a lovely long list I have now! You should write a list of things you enjoy beginning with the same letter.

BEN:     Must I?

ME:     It'll be fun.

BEN:     Will it?

* * * * * * * *

ME:     Guess what I've just done!

BEN:     Made another list?

ME:     I accidentally put Celebrity Weekly in the fridge.

BEN:     Was Peter Andre looking too hot on the cover?

ME:     Yes (smiling). If I put the mag in the oven and warm it up, will we have mag pie?

WE LAUGH

1.00 p.m.

ME: It was wonderful, watching snowflakes falling last night. I was hoping to wake up to a winter wonderland but there's not a single snowflake to be seen today.

BEN: Never mind, have a gaze at the hills around our valley instead. They're still white with snow.

ME: This will be my last winter to enjoy the hills. I'll make the most of them before my view is blocked by a wall of brick, and I'll feel imprisoned forever. And I won't be able to watch children build snowmen in the car park, and gaze at the snowmen, looking so still and eerie in the moonlight and –

BEN: Camomile tea?

ME: A large whisky would be better.

BEN: But you don't like whisky, you only fancy it when you have a bad cold.

ME: I know, but great disappointment feels like going down with something horrible, don't you think?

BEN: Yes dear, I think we have a bottle of Glenfiddich in the back of a cupboard.

ME: It's OK (smiling), bit early in the day! Especially for spirits. Unless you're watching *Most Haunted*. I just like the thought of a glass of Scottish golden liquid calming my mind and warming my body, like glowing logs in a fireplace. And making me feel merry as a *very merry* Christmas.

BEN: How about just a wee dram in a glass with a tartan pattern and golden tinsel wrapped around it?

ME: Sounds fun (giggling).

BEN: I'll join you!

\* \* \* \* \* \* \* \*

BEN: Fancy another wee dram lassie?

ME: That'll be bonny laddie. I feel Christmassy now!

BEN: And it's Sunday, so we can savour the silence on the building site.

ME: *Silent site*
*Holy site*

BEN: *The whisky in my glass is bright*

ME: *Outside the weather is sunny but cold*

BEN: *And the age of this whisky is old*

ME: *We'll dose in heavenly peace*

BEN: *Heavenly, heavenly peace*

WE LAUGH

ME: All I can hear is the sound of the crows. Tomorrow the metal beasties will wake up and start growling at each other again.

BEN: And the workmen will bark at each other, with a lot

of **F** words thrown in!

ME:    I'm counting my blessings that I've had my sight all these years to enjoy the view of the hills and trees.

*I love the hills and trees*

BEN:   *Sprouts, broccoli and peas*

ME:    *So glad I have my sight*

BEN:   *To see the crows in flight*

ME:    *I loved to the watch snowmen*

BEN:   *In the middle of the night*

ME:    I wonder what the crows are thinking as they strut about on the rubble, looking like old men in black suits, with beaky noses, their hands behind their backs.

BEN:   They'll be enjoying the peace today, quiet as the grave.

ME:    They do look so black and mournful.

BEN:   Look at the hills, the sun is making them dazzling white.

ME:    *The snow was very light*
       *In the middle of the night*
       *But now in the garden*
       *There's no snowflake in sight*

BEN:   *And my clothes are getting tight*

ME:        *When you leave turn out the light*

WE LAUGH

## Monday 4th

9.16 a.m.

ME:        Did you make your list?

BEN:     List?

ME:        Of things you enjoy beginning with the same letter.

BEN:     I did.

ME:        As Elizabeth Bennet would say in *Pride and Prejudice* – I am all astonishment! Do read it out to me kind sir, I would be most obliged.

BEN:     **M**usic
             **M**etal string guitars
             **M**aking money from music
             **M**inestrone soup
             **M**andarins

ME:        Marvellous! Great list. Fun isn't it.

BEN:     Most fun I've had for ages.

ME:        You'll find new words will just pop into your head when you least expect it.

BEN:     I'll look forward to that.

10.07 a.m.  *CLITTER, CLATTER! CLITTER, CLATTER!* of caterpillar tracks on the building site. I don't enjoy the
sound of caterpillar tracks, but I do love big hairy
caterpillars and will add them to my list.

10.08 a.m.  I watch one of the metal beasties balancing precar-
iously on top of a mound, very near our house, at the
same level as our bedroom window. Ben walks into
the room.

ME:  I've added caterpillars to my list – the big hairy ones.

BEN:  That's nice.

ME:  I'm tempted to give the driver of that digger a little
wave, the big hairy one. Look how close he is to our
window, he'll be able to see me.

BEN:  Not a good idea dear, he looks like he could tip backwards at any moment. Will you add him to your
list?

ME:  No dear. There's another workman doing the same
thing at the far end of the site, they bring to mind
scary rides at a funfair.

BEN:  Yeah.

ME:  The snow is melting away on the hills now, I want
them to stay white for longer.

BEN:  You have your colourful flowers to enjoy.

ME:  True! I've never seen hyacinth in a bunch of flowers.
The soft blue with the white tulips, yellow daffs,
and a red rose is a lovely combination. A splash of

springtime, to keep me inspired to continue with my –

BEN: Red, yellow, green and Prussian blue, spooky cat with the Mona Lisa eyes.

ME: And I'm looking forward to *Coronation Street* tonight, should be entertaining. Jenny has a meltdown.

BEN: Like the snow on the hills.

ME: There's a Swedish comedy film on later that I fancy watching because of the strange, long title – *The Pigeon Sat on a Branch Reflecting on Existence*. But I can't because it's got sub-titles – they're so tiring.

BEN: There's a good *Agatha Christie's Poirot* on at nine, you like him.

ME: So do you. You should add *murder mysteries* to your list! And I've thought of two more words – *magic* tricks and *malt* loaf, you love fresh malt loaf and a good magic trick.

BEN: Why didn't I think of that? (hand on forehead).

ME: There's a thriller on – *Paint by Murder*. I read it as *Painting by Murders*. I think that's not just because of my M.E. eyeballs. The small print of what my painting by numbers should look like when completed, has what looks like three blood red drips, dribbling from the top of the painting. Gives the painting a *Midsomer Murders* feel – you know, in the break for ads when they show blood dripping down the lettering, very sinister.

BEN: Yeah. So that's why you've painted one drip purple and another one turquoise.

ME: You noticed!

\* \* \* \* \* \* \* \* \*

6.35 p.m. Ben cooked a delicious meal of butter beans, Quorn, green beans and mushrooms on a bed of rice. Half-way through the meal I found myself mixing the rice with the vegetables, beans and Quorn, and making little mounds, then shaping them by scooping away with my fork.

BEN: I think the work on the site is getting to you dear.

ME: But I'm enjoying *demolishing* your delicious dinner.

BEN: Glad to hear it.

ME: You should add *making* a delicious *meal* to your list. And you like an after dinner *mint* after an Indian meal with one of your *mates*.

BEN: The fun never ends.

## Tuesday 5th

9.02 a.m. I plod into the kitchen after feeding my menagerie, wearing my fluffy white dressing gown and white wellies with purple and turquoise butterfly design.

BEN: You look nice in your festival wellies – like a snow-man at the Glastonbury music festival.

ME: I'll take that as a compliment. Oh, compliment! Another thing beginning with **C** that I enjoy. Have you thought of any more words to add to your list?

BEN: Can't say I have.

ME: You love cooking with *mushrooms* so that's another one.

BEN: So it is.

ME: Can you help me get my wellies off please.

BEN: Yep. Last time you wore these to a festival, I saw a few women admiring them.

ME: I didn't notice!.... I don't think I've ever worn anything that's been the envy of other women (big smile). Our new neighbour may have been admiring them just now, I saw her watching me from her window.... Heard you chatting to her the other day, she seems nice.

BEN: Yeah. She's divorced and got a little girl. Think she may have bought the house.

ME: I wondered how long it would take the landlady of number eight to get fed up with one problem tenant after another. Lets hope we'll get some peace now, with a nice quiet neighbour...... They cheer me up!

BEN: Quiet neighbours or your wellies?

ME: Both! And when the estate is built, things should be even better by next winter. No more shaking house, making the saucepans clatter on the cooker.

Is this really happening?

*The saucepans clatter*
*And raindrops splatter*
*But I'm not so bothered anymore*

BEN: *It doesn't really matter!*

ME: Looking at the mustard coloured paint for my feline masterpiece, reminds me, I forgot to ask you to get mustard. You love a nice hot mustard.

BEN: Don't tell me, another one for my list... I've thought of one! I like nice big *melons*.

ME: See, told you it would be fun.

BEN: When I'm in town I'll pop into Sainsbury's.

ME: Can you get some soups. I feel better in Winter when we have a nice stock of soups in the cupboard. And another loaf for the freezer would be good. Just in case we get more snow.

BEN: Wishful thinking again dear. Text me if you think of anything else after I've gone.

\* \* \* \* \* \* \* \*

1.45 p.m. I noticed my yellow daffodils were opening to reveal orangey bits in the middle.

I sent Ben a text:

JAFFA CAKES PLZ

## Wednesday 6th

9.20 a.m.  *CRASH!..... SMASHING GLASS!.....* Coming from the sitting room. I'm in the bedroom doing a little workmen-watching, while I wait for today's episode of *Time Team* (Tony and his team will be excavating a Stone Age site on the South Downs). I hurry to the top of the stairs and call down to Ben.

ME:  What on earth was that noise!? Are you OK?

BEN:  FINE!... (*Rumble.... rumble..... rumble..... crash..... clattering noise*). It's OK, a saucepan fell off the washing machine on spin... Hang on, I'm in the kitchen – will investigate the front room....... A picture fell off the wall and smashed into the fireplace.

ME:  I'm not surprised, I *knew* it would happen again. The house has been shaking so much this week, the clip frames have been rattling like mad on the walls.

BEN:  I'll clear up the mess before little paws tread on glass.

ME:  Thanks..... Maybe we should take all the pictures down until work on the site is completed.

BEN:  Yeah.

9.23 a.m.  **BANG!** Coming from the bathroom..... My turn to investigate......... Diamanda gallops out of the room looking alarmed......... There's a glass tumbler in the bath, surprisingly not broken – I rescued a moth, using it last night. Diamanda must have been trying to catch another one, because I spot a large moth with a partly frayed wing on the window pane. Before I can rescue it, the frightened creature flutters down onto the window ledge, then falls down a gap into the dark, dusty, cobwebby world of under-the-bath.

9.24 a.m.     ***Crack!... Crack!.... CRACK!...*** Ben calls to me, from downstairs.

BEN:          You OK dear?

ME:           No worries! I've just removed the side panel off the bath for a moth rescue mission.

BEN:          What are you like.

9.26 a.m.

ME:           Moth mission accomplished.

9.31 a.m.     I slurp a calming cuppa and nibble on a comforting Jaffa cake (with the lovely orangey bit in the middle), then feel inspired to paint an orangey bit in the middle of my painting, and maybe a chocolate and sponge coloured bit too. I'll take the opportunity, when the workmen are at lunch and the house isn't shaking, making my paint strokes go all wibbly-wobbly.

9.32 a.m.     An Elvis Presley song pops into my head and I sing to myself.

              *Well my hands are shaky and my knees are weak*
              *I can't seem to stand on my own two feet*
              *Who do you thank when you have such luck*
              *I'm in love*
              *I'm all shook up*

**10.02 p.m.**

ME: I fancy peas and quiet for dinner tonight.

BEN: I think we have some in the freezer (laughing).

ME: I want peas on earth, and good dill for all men too.

BEN: Are you feeling alright?

ME: My brain's just a little shaken......... as Elvis would sing, I'm all shook up.

BEN: What's dill?

ME: A herb of the parsley family.

BEN: Oh, right. And one of the characters in the sixties children's programme, *The Herbs*.

ME: Yes, I recall Dill the dog, the very friendly lion called Parsley, and Rosemary who looked and spoke like one of the characters in present day *Coronation Street* – Audrey Roberts.

\* \* \* \* \* \* \* \*

**11.45 p.m.** There's a workman in his digger, on top of a mound of rubble, quite near our house. The digger is stationary and he's shouting at a man at the foot of the mound. I open the window to hear what he is saying because I'm feeling super-nosey today.

**11.51 p.m.**

ME: Oh God, I'm so embarrassed!

BEN:     Why, what have you done now?

ME:      I was being nosey, trying to hear what a workman was shouting about, when suddenly, him and his workmate turned and looked *straight at me*. Then I realised I was leaning forward at the window, revealing more than I should, and quickly covered myself up.

BEN:     That may have been the highlight of their day!

ME:      They didn't look happy, just more annoyed.

BEN:     Maybe they wanted you to reveal more (laughing).

ME:      That's not going to happen (giggling). I can happily gaze at Tony and his jolly band of archaeologists on *Time Team* in a minute – they won't notice! They'll be too busy excavating a Stone Age site in our part of the country today, then a medieval chapel dedicated to Edward the Confessor. I wonder what he confessed to.

BEN:     No idea. I'll Google it.

ME:      I'll watch *Digging Up Britain's Past* tonight, after we've enjoyed peas and quiet for dinner – we could have peas and quiche!

BEN:     Anything you say dear.

ME:      *Coronation Street* should be good, Rita is going to thwart Brian and Kathy's announcement – that's probably about The Kabin. Can't wait!

2.10 p.m.

BEN: Edward the Confessor was one of the last Anglo-Saxon kings of England. Usually considered the last king of the House of Wessex, he ruled from ten forty-two to ten sixty-six.

ME: Ten sixty-six, the Battle of Hastings. I have a funny story about that – well it's not *that* funny, but at the time I thought it was.

BEN: Were you at the battle in a past life dear?

ME: No, but I believe I have an ancestor who fought with William the Conqueror. Anyway, I was in Thornton's. This was before I got M.E. Which does seem like a past life now.

BEN: *YOU?*..... In a shop *full of CHOCOLATES*?

ME: It *was Christmas* and Thornton's do a *wonderful*, delicious selection of Christmas chocolatey gifts.

BEN: And there's chocolate on the counter for you to sample.

ME: True. Anyway, I was at the counter paying for my purchases, and the assistant said it cost ten sixty-six. So I said, Battle of Hastings, and she stared at me as if I were a nutter, and I almost spat out my nutty chocolate-treat-from-the-counter. Wish you'd you'd been there, you'd have laughed too. Anyway, do continue.

BEN: Edward's nickname reflects the traditional image of him as unworldly and pious. Confessor reflects his reputation as a saint who did not suffer martyrdom, as opposed to his uncle, King Edward the Martyr.

ME: Thank you. I must confess I feel better for knowing that.

## Thursday 7th

I woke up in the night after a nightmare – the house was constantly shaking, and I ran from room to room trying to catch pictures and ornaments as they fell to the floor, but they fell through my hands and smashed to pieces. The windows began to crack, then shattered. As I lay on the floor, completely shattered, King Edward the Confessor appeared at a window, wearing his crown and finery, to confess it was all his fault. Then the assistant from Thornton's appeared, wearing a milk chocolate brown cloak, and said she knew nothing about what was going on or the Battle of Hastings.

9.17 a.m. I told Ben about my nightmare.

BEN: Sounds amusing, and chilling.

ME: It was. Freezing winds blew in from the windows without panes. So the assistant from Thornton's offered me her cloak and a hot chocolate, but the cloak blew away and the hot chocolate turned freezing cold. Then –

BEN: Would you like a nice hot camomile tea dear?

ME: Yes please.

10.15 a.m.

ME: I've just been feeding the birds – the strong winds nearly blew me away.

BEN: There were gales in the night, the noise woke me up (we yawn in unison).

ME: I remember waking up to hear bangs and clatters. I'd love a nice quiet and peaceful day.

BEN: You enjoyed nice quiche and peas-full dinner with tomatoes last night.

ME: I did!

\* \* \* \* \* \* \* \*

11.19 a.m. There's a drill... drill... drilling noise in the bathroom. Ben is installing the new toilet cistern he sprayed a beautiful green, that almost matches our avocado green bath and hand basin.

11.25 a.m. There's a bang... bang... banging from our neighbour at number 6. Something is being hammered on the wall.

11.30 a.m. There's a yap... yap.... yap... woof... woof... woofing at the end of our street. And a baby cries, startled by the barking and loud beeping noise as a vehicle reverses out of the building site.

11.35 a.m. Meow... meow... meow... Diamanda demands a tuna treat.

11.36 a.m. Roar... roar... roar... of a motorbike the other end of the building site.

11.37 a.m.   Clothes scream – wash me!.... Plants weep – I'm thirsty!.... The stair carpet shouts – hoover me!

11.38 a.m.   I recall mum used to say, 'No peace for the wicked' (in her lilting Irish voice). I must be very wicked for not doing enough housework.

11.39 a.m.   I will not have peas with dinner tonight – no peas for the wicked.

11.40 a.m.   I curl up under the bed covers. So tired. Is this really happening?

\* \* \* \* \* \* \* \*

12.40 p.m.   Peace at last. The workmen are on their lunch break. No more hammering from number 6 or drilling from the bathroom. No more barking dogs or crying babies, meowing cat, roaring or beeping. Plants watered. Stair carpet hoovered. Just the gentle rumbling of the washing machine. I am no longer wicked. So I can have peas with dinner if I like.

12.42 p.m.   I plan my TV viewing, with a refreshing minty cuppa.

12.43 p.m.   I plan dinner. Maybe we'll have veggie sausages, with broccoli and potatoes. And minty peas.

12.44 p.m.   Watching *Time Team*. Tony and his team are in Wales, searching for the remains of a Roman town with the help of geophysics. Later they'll be in Scotland excavating an Iron Age stone tower. I wish they were digging opposite our house. I could invite them in from the cold for a cuppa and slice of coffee and walnut cake. And they could tell me stories of past digs.

12.45 p.m.   That's a nice daydream but I notice, *in reality* two programmes this week will be in *our town!*

12.46 p.m.   Two programmes! The most excited I've felt since a really good storyline in *Coronation Street*.

2.03 p.m.

ME:   You know Peter Andre was in our town a few years ago, doing his *60 Minute Makeover*, then Phil and Kirstie were only a few streets away, presenting *Location, Location, Location?*

BEN:   Yeah.

ME:   Well, I see in TV Weekly, two more programmes will be in our town this week. One this afternoon and one tomorrow night. Have a guess which ones.

BEN:   Must I?

ME:   Just have a few guesses. I'll give you a clue. One is a programme I often watch in the evenings, and one I don't like, in the day, because it's boring people being critical. But I'll watch it tomorrow because it's in our town.

BEN:   It's not *Coronation Street*, that's up north. Or *Doc Martin* in the West Country. Is it a murder mystery?

ME:   No.

BEN:      Need another clue.

ME:      The one in the evening is about buildings. The one in the day is probably set in a house like the ones round the corner in Hale Street – judging by the odd bits of programme I've watched in moments of mad boredom, when there's nothing else on.

BEN:      *House Doctor*? *Building The Dream*?

ME:      No, but close (smiling because I'm having fun).

BEN:      *Grand Designs*?

ME:      *YES!*... That's the evening one.

BEN:      Phew..... can't think of the second one.

ME:      It's *Four In A Bed*. Couples rate how good other couple's B&B's are. The name of the B&B in tomorrow's programme reminds me of you.

BEN:      Ben's B&B?

ME:      Windy Bottom B&B!

BEN:      Maybe they serve a lot of greens with breakfast.

ME:      Eggs Florentine with piles of spinach and a side dish of cabbage.

## WE LAUGH

3.10 p.m.    Staring out of the bedroom window, I watch a workman climb down from a JCB. As he does this I notice his strong manly hands, and his jeans come down at the back revealing quite a lot of flesh, so I'm tempted to open the window and call out, 'Nice bum!'

3.11 p.m.    No peas for the wicked for me tonight. But think, as Ben is out for the evening, will have an evening breakfast of poached eggs on muffins, with steamed baby spinach and asparagus tips. What shall I call it? Very late brunch?... No.... An *evenfast?* No, that sounds religious – a cross between Evensong and a time of fasting. And singing on an empty stomach is no fun. I will call it Eggs Florentine with asparagus, evening delight.

3.30 p.m.    I really fancy Eggs Florentine and vegetable delight now. Can't stop thinking about it. So shall I change the name?... Yes... Eggs Florentine with asparagus, afternoon delight. And peas, because I haven't been *that* wicked.

3.31 p.m.    Feel too tired at the moment to prepare the meal. And if I do, I'll have to cook extra for Ben because the smell of cooking will make him hungry (and will spoil his appetite for the meal with his mate). Although on second thoughts, whatever he eats, at whatever time, his appetite *NEVER* seems to be spoilt.

3.32 p.m.    But after all the food preparation and cooking I'll be too tired to eat.

4.00 p.m.    I dip lightly toasted soldiers into thick creamy egg yolk, while watching a cook teaching vegan recipes in France, in *A New Life in The Sun,* on Channel 4.

ME:    Are you enjoying your egg and soldiers?

BEN:    Parfait!

## Friday 8th

1.20 p.m.  After a most enjoyable episode of *Time Team* (today they may not have been in our town, but they were in a county next to ours – Sussex), I sat and did a little watch-the-workmen-working, to rest my eyes. As soon as I peered out of the window I saw the man with the loose jeans and nice hands, standing on top of a mound of rubble, close to our window, staring *right at me*. I wondered if I should smile, give him a friendly wave, or mouth, 'Nice bum'. I felt a little wicked, but did what a cat does when it's embarrassed – I scratched my ear and quickly looked away with an I'm-not-embarrassed-just-got-a-sudden-itch-behind-my-right-ear expression. Then I stroked Diamanda in an I'm-just-stroking-my-cat-in-the-window way.

2.05 p.m.  I snooze to the snooker, enjoying the gentle click-clack and tip-tap sound, occasional ripple of applause, and running commentary........... *he hit the red a little too thick........ deciding which side of the blue........ knock-on effect........ below the black...... wonderful shot.......... if he pots the yellow, green and blue........... more top spin............. a wee bit too much pace.*

2.20 p.m.  I can't help noticing the man leaning across the snooker table has a nice wee bum. That's twice I've been wicked today.

2.21 p.m.  Watching balls rolling around on a snooker table is making me (no, not have wicked thoughts) want to continue painting a wee bit more of my cat portrait, inspired by the colours.

2.22 p.m.    *Another miss....... knocks the black to the cushion.... he doesn't need two awkward reds either side of the cushion.*

2.23 p.m.    Will paint more black either side of some of the red bits on the cat's forehead. Maybe the odd green and blue bits too, until I get tired – the house isn't shaking this afternoon, so I'll have a fairly steady hand.

3.14 p.m.    Time for another snooze with the snooker....... *The pink goes down....... behind the brown......... hits a wee bit too hard........ red over the middle pocket ......... wonderful shot!......... see you in a wee while.*

3.16p.m.     I've drifted off to sleep, to dream of workmen on the building site playing snooker with spades and diggers – knocking yellow, pink, blue, green, yellow, brown and red hard hats into deep holes in the four corners of the site........ Then after a while, the brown earth on the site becomes the green (as grass grows) of a snooker table and the workmen are kicking around footballs, all the colours of snooker balls – aiming to pot them into the six holes around the edge of the site.

5.10 p.m.

BEN:         I'll cook tonight. What do you fancy?

ME:          Veggie Quorn balls, rolling around on a bed of green salad, with green beans or asparagus and spinach. But no peas for the wicked.

## Saturday 9th

9.10 a.m.   As I wandered into the garden to feed the wildlife, I was *almost* blown away by the wind again, but *completely* blown away by the delicate beauty of my robin who perched near to me, bobbing happily.

10.00 a.m.   I watched a rather chunky, ugly workman pace about, ranting angrily into his mobile phone. As he did so, he gave certain parts of his anatomy, kept in baggy grey, rather grubby sweatpants, a good scratch. Then one of his workmates relieved himself in a place he thought no-one could see him. But I could. I didn't actually *see* his private parts, but still felt a bit wicked again for witnessing all these goings on.

11.25 a.m.

BEN:   Three catalogues have arrived for you dear.

ME:   Oh, goody. Time to stop being a wicked-workmen-watcher and be an angelic catalogue peruser.

BEN:   Who is wicked? The workmen or you?

* * * * * * * *

11.30 a.m.

ME:   Ooh, there's some really nice colouring books in this gift catalogue. Enchanting fairies, unicorns, flowers and butterflies. But I'm up to my eyes with –

BEN:   Painting the cat with the spooky eyes, that are still following me around the room.

ME:   There's some really good jigsaw puzzles too. *Fantasy toy shop, National Park, Mad Catter's Tea Party.*

BEN:      Don't you mean Mad Hatter's Tea Party?

ME:      No (giggling), it's lots of crazy cats, similar to the crazy cats jigsaw puzzle I did years ago in a potting shed (the cats were in a potting shed, not me), but these cats are at a tea party, and one is wearing a top hat. The detail is wonderful but –

BEN:      You've got enough detail to work on, coping with the crazy looking cat in your spooky cat painting.

* * * * * * * *

1.50 p.m.      *KNOCK! KNOCK! KNOCK!* Ben opens the front door to be greeted by a cheerful delivery man.

BEN:      Cheers mate! Can't remember what it is.

MAN:      That's what ninety-five percent of my customers say. Or they want to know what it is!

THEY LAUGH

ME:      Is it another *round-tuit*? So you can get around to it. Have you remembered what it is?

BEN:      No (opening well wrapped parcel).

ME:      Oh (looking at the picture on the box) looks like an iron.

BEN:      It's a palm sander.

ME:      So you'll be getting *around to it* on the front door.

BEN:       When the weather is better.

ME:        Lovely. I'd like it to be painted apple green because we live in Orchard Street, and in memory of the orchard that was once where a new housing estate is going to be.

BEN:       Anything you say dear.

ME:        Do you remember me saying, if we lived in Quality Street I'd like a purple front door, with a gold knocker and letter box. And the window frames painted Quality Street wrapper red and green.

BEN:       I do. And feel most fortunate we don't live in Quality Street.

## Sunday 10th

ME:        I've been *seeing things* on the building site, my eyes have been playing tricks on me. You'll never guess what I saw.

BEN:       Not in a million years.

ME:        A huge black panther crouching by the fence, near a pile of planks of wood – come and look!

BEN:       Must I?

ME:        It'll make you smile.

                              * * * * * * * *

BEN:       Oh, yeah. Does look a bit cat like (smiling). It's just a sheet of black plastic covering something.

ME: The wind and rain is making it appear the cat's hind quarters are moving, ready to pounce on a workman.

BEN: Yeah!

ME: Over the other side I thought I saw a pond with four white ducks swimming on it. Then I put my distance glasses on and realised –

BEN: It's a large sheet of black plastic rippling in the wind and rain, held down with four white bricks (smiling again).

ME: I wish the site was going to be an animal or bird sanctuary. So I could sit and watch the animals or birds all day (big sigh).

BEN: You have your little menagerie in the garden.

ME: That I have, to be sure! And this little one (stroking Diamanda's tiny head, along her silky back and down to her beautiful furry tail ending).

BEN: This afternoon I'm going to record the ending of some music for a backing track I've been working on.

ME: OK. I'll be as quiet as a sleeping black cat. I'll sail around the house, silently as white ducks on a pond. And softly stroke liquid onto canvas, without a sound.

\* \* \* \* \* \* \* \*

2.07 p.m. WHY is it? *Why, why, why?* When you are making

the effort to be quiet, you make a lot of noise? You send a saucepan *CRASHING* to the floor, when all you are doing is making a cuppa.

2.20 p.m.   You accidentally knock over a paper cup of water that you've been rinsing your paintbrush in, and the paint you've been using is black, red and blue, so the water is a horrible muddy grey, and it's only a small paper cup but the water seems to splash everywhere – onto important paper work, the pretty pink envelope of a birthday card you've just stamped and addressed, ready to post (making the writing blurry), and the cover of TV Weekly – making it soggy and the faces of Brian and Kathy of *Coronation Street* more miserable. And the pages are stuck together. And you forget you are being quiet. And say a rude word. LOUDLY.

2.26 p.m.   And your cat, who sleeps a lot in the afternoon, decides to *THUNDER* up and down the stairs, then jumps onto the coffee table, knocking over some paperwork with half a mug of cold coffee sitting on top, sending envelopes and letters flying everywhere and the mug *SMASHING* into the fireplace.

2.30 p.m.   You settle down to watch a vintage sit-com with your cat. It's one of your favourite episodes of *The Good Life*, where Margo and Jerry have to spend Christmas with Tom and Barbara. They are pulling crackers made out of newspaper, and they say 'Bang,' and you laugh. OUT LOUD.

2.31 p.m.

ME:        So sorry about the noise.

BEN: I'll finish my recording when you've gone to bed, and Diamanda is snoring in her favourite box.

## Monday 11th

10.03 a.m. The workmen have returned to the building site, making more noise than usual. Radio 1 blaring out rock music. Lots of shouting. Swearing. Sweating. Scratching of parts kept in sweatpants. Stomping in the mud. Pulling lengths of pipework in the cold, and pulling faces, when they'd rather be in the pub where Pamela the barmaid is pulling pints in the warm.

They've dug about six feet down into the site now, and when work starts on the foundations, I'll imagine I'm watching *Grand Designs* live – but it will have to be without the lovely Kevin McCloud telling me what materials are being used and the challenges faced during construction, while lively music is played in the background, making it all the more entertaining.

Then at the end of the programme, there's the heavenly music – a waltz melody with lilting angelical voices, and up-lifting harp – because people who build their own grand designs are a little God-like, creating their own worlds, and they have the patience of a saint to endure the challenges – design problems, unexpected costs, and sometimes being let down by builders, banks, or the weather. Or if they are very unlucky, all three.

ME: The workmen are listening to *rock* music while they dig up *rocks,* that's quite funny!

BEN: Very amusing. Are they listening to the seventies

Is this really happening?

band *Mud* too.

\* \* \* \* \* \* \* \*

ME:     I've been *seeing creatures* on the building site again.

BEN:    A hippo wallowing in the mud?

ME:     *Mud, mud, glorious mud*
        *Nothing quite like it for cooling the blood*

BEN:    *So follow me follow*
        *Down to the hollow*

ME:     *And there we will wallow*

BEN:    *In glorious, glorious*

ME:     *Mud!*
                    WE LAUGH

ME:     We're together for better or verse.

BEN:    What creatures have you been *seeing*?

ME:     A digger that looks like a great big dinosaur, drinking at a watering hole.

BEN:    Great.

ME:     And an enormous brown snake slithering through the mud, then –

BEN:    You put your glasses on and realised it was piping being pulled through mud by a workman who was out of view.

ME:     For a second it was quite exciting (yawning).

BEN:    I expect you wish Tony and his team of archaeologists were out there, on one of their digs.

ME:     It would be brilliant! After a hard day's digging and painstaking picking, scraping and everything; they could pop into our house with little Tupperware boxes full of interesting finds, like Roman coins, pieces of pottery and mosaic, and *whole* skeletons! And I could very carefully wash the finds in our kitchen sink and bath, then lay them gently on towels, on our bed to dry. You wouldn't mind helping me would you.

BEN:    No, it would be fun, a bunch of old skeletons lying on our bed. Very nice.

ME:     We could give them tea and cake.

BEN:    To fatten up the skeletons?

ME:     Very funny. After refreshments, Tony could tell us stories of their most exciting finds in England, Scotland and Wales. And later we could dress in medieval costumes, hired from our local fancy dress shop in Union Street, and cook them a mini-medieval banquet. It would have to be a veggie banquet, but they wouldn't notice because they'd be merry on beer and wine. And it wouldn't matter how merry they got because they'd have comfy camper vans on the site to sleep in at night. You could play medieval songs on your guitar and we'd all sing along. Could you find one or two on the internet? I'd like to sing some today for fun. I could make up melodies, if they are not well known.

BEN: Certainly dear.

ME: We'd have so much fun singing with Tony and his team, he would invite us to watch their next dig on a remote island off the coast of Scotland. We could be their caterers and entertainment. And when we're not catering or entertaining, I could paint watercolours or sketch the island and wildlife. Although, knowing me, before we left, I'd be so busy thinking about packing lots of warm clothing, and reminding you to pack lots of warm clothing, and thinking about what warming, energy giving food to take to cater for the hard working archaeologists, I'd forget to pack my pencils, paints and sketch pads. You could take photographs of the beautiful island and wildlife because you love taking photos. And walk around the island and explore because you love walking and exploring. And if you were bored, you could help out with a bit of archaeological work. I used to be an amateur archaeologist, so I could advise you and we could work together, when I had a bit of energy. It would be exciting!

BEN: I'm sure it would.

\* \* \* \* \* \* \* \*

BEN: Here you are, I've printed out some songs for you.

ME: Oh goody..... Ah, the cuckoo song. Spelt with a **u** at the end.

*Summer is icumin in,*
*Loude sing cuckou!*
*Groweth seed and bloweth mead,*
*And springeth the wode now.*

*Sing cuckou!*

BEN:  She's off!

## Tuesday 12th

1.05 p.m.

ME:  *Most Haunted* was good just now. Yvette and her team were doing a seance in a haunted pub, dating back centuries, with a priest hole. Doors opened by themselves and objects were thrown. The creepiest bit was the voices of children being heard in a corridor. Anyway, I was feeling a bit spooked and jumpy –

BEN:  Like you always are, halfway through the programme.

ME:  When, at the same moment as the seance table shook violently, our house shook violently too and –

BEN:  There's more?

ME:  A barrel in the pub cellar started rolling across the floor by itself – they had cameras filming it. The sound it made on the concrete floor was similar to a sound on the building site.

BEN:  That sounds a barrel of fun.

ME:  And when Yvette's team were knocking on a boarded-up fireplace, hoping for a response, there was a hammering from next door.

BEN:  Calming camomile tea dear?

3.05 p.m.

ME:      Phew, the repeat of *Coronation Street* was wonderfully creepy too today. Shona discovered someone had filmed her while she slept. And Carla found Roy sleepwalking. Have you ever sleepwalked?

BEN:    No.

ME:      Me neither. But I've known people who have. The thought is quite scary.

BEN:    Seen any more creepy creatures on the building site?

ME:      Not today. But there's a sheet of flat, plastic looking stuff. It's brown with square shaped mouldings like a giant bar of Cadbury's milk chocolate. Next to it there's a triangular mound of earth with white bits in it, like a ten foot high Toblerone.

BEN:    So there may be Toblerone or a Cadbury's choc bar on the shopping list?

ME:      Maybe Toblerone. I saw Joey eating a supersized one on *Friends*. It looked very tasty.

BEN:    *Greatest Chocolate Ads of All Time* is on tonight. Don't think you should watch it.

ME:      I'm already recalling some of the songs for the ads.

          *Only the crumbliest, flakiest chocolate*

BEN:    *Tastes like chocolate never tasted before*

ME:      *A Mars a day*

BEN:    *Helps you work rest and play*

ME:     *The milky bar kid is strong and tough*
        *And only the best is good enough*

BEN:    *The creamiest milk, the whitest bar* – we'd better
        stop, I'm craving chocolate now.

ME:     Do you remember the advert for Toblerone, with
        the triangular bees?...... Don't worry, I won't sing
        the song!

BEN:    I'm off into town. I won't ask you to text if you think
        any treats you fancy. Could be a very long list.

                        WE LAUGH

3.15 p.m.   I put the kettle on, singing to myself.

            *Triangular chocolate from triangular trees*
            *La, la, la, la, triangular bees*
            *And oh Mr Confectioner please*
            *Give me Toblerone*

3.16 p.m.   I put some nuts out for the birds, singing to them.

            *Everyone's a fruit and nutcase*
            *Crazy for those Cadbury's nuts and raisins*

3.18 p.m.   I put my feet up and sing to Diamanda.

            *When you put your feet up*
            *What's the bar you eat up*
            *City gents of consequence*
            *And men who dig the street up*

3.20 p.m.  I took a trip down chocolatey memory lane, and surprised myself by remembering lots of ads and the slogans... *Who knows the secrets of the Black Magic box..... Roses grow on you...... If you love someone, give them your last Rolo..... Bounty, a taste of paradise....... Have a break, have a Kit-Kat.... Take it easy with Cadbury's Caramel.*

3.30 p.m.  I watch a man climbing into a large truck, and recall the man in an ad, going to all sorts of lengths to deliver a box of chocolates to a lady........ *And all because the lady loves Milk Tray.*

3.40 p.m.  I'm in the bathroom washing my hands, singing to my plants.

*A finger of fudge is just enough to give your kids a treat*

*La, la, la, la, la, la, la, la, it's very small and neat*

4.00 p.m.  Ben returns home with a *round-tuit*.

BEN:  I *know* what you've been doing, and I *know* if you don't have chocolate very soon you will die.

ME:  I don't *know* what you mean (grinning).

BEN:  Close your eyes and open your paws.

ME:  Lovely! (opening eyes). I haven't had one of these since I was little. It was in a Christmas stocking.

8.05 p.m.  I'm watching *Grand Designs*. As bricks are being broken up, I snap a triangular shaped piece off my chocolatey treat.

8.06 p.m.    I hum the little tune about triangular trees and triangular bees.

## Wednesday 13th

2.01 p.m.

ME:    I used to be a pantomime horse – I quit while I was a head.

BEN:    What are you like.

ME:    I used to be a surgeon – I raised a few eyebrows.

BEN:    Have you been watching *Live at the Apollo*?

ME:    I have. And now I'm going to snooze to the snooker while you get around to it with your *round-tuit*.

2.04 p.m.    I'm wishing I hadn't watched the programme about chocolate ads. I can't help imagining the snooker balls are big shiny chocolates, because I recall seeing snooker ball shaped chocolates in a triangular box, in ACE Christmas gift catalogue last Christmas.

2.05 p.m.    *He's potted the lemon dream............ Just missed the mint.......... There goes the toffee treat............ The timing has got to be perfect..... The vanilla perfection just taps the raspberry romance........... Difficult to hit full on............ He's potted another strawberry sensation...... Nicely played!*

2.28 p.m.    I doze off, to dream of the workmen on the building site taking a break with giant KitKats. As well as eating them, they put some KitKat fingers aside to use as fence posts. One man breaks a square off the huge bar of Cadbury's chocolate (that I thought I saw on the site yesterday) with a hammer.

2.34 p.m.  A purple, shiny, Cadbury's wrapper (the size of a double bed sheet) flutters away in the wind.

2.35 p.m.  I awake with a start. Shiny, purple chocolate wrapper! Just remembered! I meant to make a Valentine's Day card for Ben using the *Quality Street* wrappers I saved from Christmas indulgence. I always make him a card. And it's Valentine's Day tomorrow!

2.36 p.m.  The snooker audience are applauding – I imagine they are applauding me – she remembered just in time!

2.41 p.m.  I'll just snooze a little longer.......... *Double red to the left of the black......... The green remains in a safe position......... Needs to get past the blue........ Not enough distance between the reds....... Keen to get the ball next to the pink........ Behind the brown.*

2.46 p.m.  Brown! Chocolate brown! Must find *Quality Street* wrappers, black card, nail scissors, glue, creative energy, and make card while Ben is busy getting around to it.

2.51 p.m.  Kettle on.

2.56 p.m.  Creative head on (with the help of Toblerone).

3.01 p.m.  Smile on face as I cut out little heart shapes from shiny, gold, purple, red and pink sweet wrappers.

3.06 p.m.  Diamanda sits on the ready-to-stick-on-black-card heart shapes, with a sweet-cat-smile on her little black whiskery face.

3.11 p.m.     I don't have the heart to move her, she's just warming them up, and flattening them nicely for me.

## Thursday 14th

8.00 a.m.     All was quiet on the building site front. Wonderfully quiet and peaceful. Our house, blissfully still.

8.05 a.m.     The sunrise shone loving reds, golds and pinks over our town, warming the rooftops.

8.06 a.m.     Lovers in love kissed the day good morning.

8.07 a.m.     I dreamily watched the shadows of flying crows ripple over mounds of earth on the site, like hot chocolate sauce pouring over chocolate gateau.

8.21 a.m.     A Cadbury's Flake awaited me in the kitchen when I sleepily plodded downstairs to switch the kettle on for my morning minty cuppa. Ben must have remembered the Flake advert was my favourite one, with the girl sitting in a cornfield, painting a watercolour and blissfully enjoying the crumbliest flakiest chocolate. There was a box of Milk Tray too – another one of my favourite adverts. *And all because the lady loves.....*

8.22 a.m.     I opened a marshmallow pink envelope and my heart melted like vanilla ice cream on very-hot-out-of-the-oven apple pie, when I took the card out and saw the photo of a kitten curled up with a puppy. It was a black and white photo, which made the little, shiny red heart between the kitten and the puppy stand out beautifully.

| | |
|---|---|
| 8.35 a.m. | Ben opened his card. |
| BEN: | Sweet card – thanks! |
| ME: | I know a good *quality* card is up your *street!* Loved your card, and I'm sure you went to great lengths to get the Milk Tray, like the man in the advert, jumping out of a helicopter and over rooftops. |
| BEN: | Of course!..... Heart-shaped veggie burgers tonight? |
| ME: | Yes please! And there's romantic comedy films on TV tonight – *Bridget Jones: The Edge of Reason* and *Valentine's Day.* Or we could watch *First Dates; Valentine's Special.* |
| BEN: | Must we dear? |

* * * * * * * *

*All you need is love. But a little chocolate now and then doesn't hurt.*

Charles Schulz

# March

**Tuesday 5th**

ME:      It's pancake day today! Shall we have pancakes tonight?

BEN:    Yeah!

ME:      You used to love *flipping* pancakes.

BEN:    Pop the ingredients on my shoppin' list.

ME:      We've got eggs, milk, lemon juice and salt. Just need the flour and honey.

BEN:    I'm dropping in to see our bee-keeping friend Rob later, so I'll pick up a jar of his honey.

ME:      It *is most deliciously* light and sweetly sweet...... I heard on Radio Kent of a woman who wanted to keep bees. She bought ten bees from a bee keeper, but when she got home, discovered she had eleven. So she rang the bee keeper to tell him and he said, 'Don't worry, it's a free bee'.

BEN:    Freebie! I'll tell that one to Rob (chuckling).

ME:      There's a mouth-watering photo in Weekly Wife of a pancake spread with Nutella and fresh berries – chocolatey sweet, nutty and little fruity. I think –

BEN:    Yes, will add to the list honey.

ME:      Wendy of Weekly Wife gives us a tip – when frying, never turn the pancake more than once.

BEN:      I'll try to remember.

ME:      She also says it's fun to flip the pancake within an inch –

BEN:      Of your life?

ME:      Of the kitchen ceiling dear. And position the pan to perfectly catch the pancake on the way down.

BEN:      Do you remember what happened last time I tried that?

ME:      No.

BEN:      One of our cats almost wore a batter jacket.

ME:      I feel some verse coming on.

> *I had a cat*
> *Her..*
> *She was mad as a hatt*
> *Er...*
> *You almost dressed her in batt*
> *Er....*
> *You said it didn't matt*
> *Er......*

But... Er.... Seriously. Flipping pancakes may not be a good idea then. And by the way, Wendy makes all sorts of suggestions for pancake toppings that we could try.

BEN:      I'm sure you're going to tell me *all* about them.... I wonder why hatters were mad.

ME:       I can tell you about that too. Mercury used to be used in the felt industry for making hats and mercury poisoning became endemic. Dementia was a common ailment among nineteenth century hat makers. Very sad.

BEN:      So that's why the hatter is mad in *Alice In Wonderland*. Or is it *Alice Through The Looking Glass?*

ME:       Not sure. I'll look on the cover of our *Alice Through The Looking Glass* DVD. That should give me a clue.

* * * * * * * *

ME:       Yes! Johnny Depp is the Mad Hatter on the cover. He was marvellously mad!...... Those crazy eyes!...... The curly, bright red hair!...... Maple syrup.

BEN:      Maple syrup? Is that the new word for mad?

ME:       It could be. Your brain must turn to treacle when you go crazy...... Maple syrup just popped into my head. Along with golden syrup, chocolate sauce, raspberries, strawberries, blueberry sauce and grated cheese – all suggestions for pancake toppings by Wendy of Weekly Wife. Do any of them appeal to your taste buds?

BEN:      I'd like hummus, cheese and chilli sauce.

ME:       Why not? If it's what takes your fancy. Add sliced tomato or a little spring onion too. Go mad!

BEN:      I think I will, I'll go maple syrup (grinning).

ME:       I've always imagined pancakes with *just* sugar and lemon, because that's what we had at home when I was little. You and I had honey and lemon last time we had em' *many moons* ago, when we first lived together.

BEN: I remember. We had honey, when we were on our lemonmoon.

ME: Lemonmoon?! (cackling). You are sounding as maple syrup as me these days. Is a lemonmoon just a rind of moon?

WE LAUGH

ME: You could have savoury pancakes, then honey and lemonmoon pancakes for afters!

BEN: *Could* life get more exciting.

＊ ＊ ＊ ＊ ＊ ＊ ＊ ＊

ME: I've had more culinary ideas for later this month.

BEN: Can't wait to hear.

ME: Have you noticed the shamrock-shaped cookies on the calendar in the kitchen, with green and white icing.

BEN: No.

ME: They are eaten on St. Patrick's Day.

BEN: When's that?

ME: The seventeenth. We used to have green cupcakes

when I was little and wear shamrock at the St Patrick's Day parades in London. We should have a green dinner.

BEN: Don't tell me. Green Tagliatelle, with green beans, peas and broccoli –

ME: Or a green cauliflower and green peppers cut into shamrock shapes.

BEN: With a creamy sauce, dyed emerald green – for the Emerald Isle?

ME: That sounds *grand,* so it does, so it does (my best Irish accent). And we could dress in green. Me, like a little pixie. You like a leprechaun.

BEN: I haven't got any green clothes, I gave my green trousers to charity. And the shirt you gave me with green leaf pattern is too tight now.

ME: You got out of that nicely!

BEN: Phew (wiping brow).

3.00 p.m.

ME: I see they're making progress on the building site with the foundations. I've tried to imagine I'm watching *Grand Designs* and I'm interested in what's going on, but it's not working. It's such a horrible sight, it makes my eyes sore looking at it.

BEN: It's a *site* for sore eyes.

ME: It is. I want to get a piece of long ribbon – yellow

ribbon to match the yellow diggers – tie it across the entrance to the site, then do a little renaming ceremony.

BEN: Cut the ribbon with your best kitchen scissors and rename the site, a-horrible-site-for-sore-eyes.

ME: And no-one would clap. But I have noticed there's a new, jolly workman who likes to sing. He may burst into song!

*Tie a yellow ribbon 'round the old oak tree*
*It's been three long years*
*Do you still want me?*
*If I don't see a ribbon 'round the old oak tree*

BEN: *I'll stay on the bus*
*Forget about us*
*Put the blame on me*
*If I don't see a ribbon 'round the old oak tree*

WE LAUGH

## Wednesday 6th

9.20 a.m.

BEN: What are you doing?

ME: Just scraping a bit of pancake off the floor.

BEN: I got a bit carried away last night.

ME: It's a good job Diamanda was in her box!

BEN:     Yeah.... They were very tasty though, the ones that ended up on a plate.

ME:      Very!......... Is that a cat crunchie or a pea-bug on the floor by the sink? I haven't got my glasses on, they slide off my nose when I bend down and forward.

BEN:     It's a dried-up pea.

ME:      Ah, thanks. Is that a spider by the fridge?

BEN:     It's a tomato stalk.

ME:      I once admired a large moth, telling it what beautiful markings it had on its wings, many shades of beige and brown.

BEN:     And it turned out to be a piece of baked potato skin, I remember.

\* \* \* \* \* \* \* \*

ME:      The daffodils you got have opened up nicely, they smell deliciously *springtimey*, and look so lovely.

BEN:     This almond milk isn't so delicious or lovely!

ME:      Yes. It tastes like........ I don't know........ old fat in a baking tray. Not that I've tasted old fat, it's more like the smell of it, if you know what I mean.

BEN:     It was a bit of a mistake, I meant to get soya milk.

ME:      Shame, it sounds so nutritious on the carton – a good source of calcium, vitamin B2 and B12 *and* D2. Low in saturated fat and naturally lactose free. I should try to make myself like it, but I can't.

BEN: It's bitter tasting.

ME: As bitter as a man whose nutty wife left him with four hungry children and a crop in the field, to bring up on his own, because she ran off with an almond farmer, with chestnut hair, and thighs that could crack walnuts.

BEN: He'd had some bad times, lived through the sad times but this time her hurtin' won't heal.

ME: She picked a fine time to leave him, Lucille.

*You picked a fine time to leave me Lucille*

BEN: *Four hungry children and a crop in the field*

ME: *I've had some bad times, lived through some sad times*

BEN: *But this time your hurtin' won't heal*

ME: *You picked a fine time to leave Lucille*

I used to sing four hundred children, instead of four hungry children. I don't know if I thought they were the correct lyrics.

WE LAUGH

3.26 p.m.

ME: The house wasn't shaking this afternoon, so I got

222

more of my cat painting done. What do you think?

BEN: Great! The eyes are more spooky and the ears are more eerie.

ME: I must pace myself more, not paint so often. It's more fatiguing than I'll admit to myself. I wonder if I'll ever finish it. My eyes are bleary from all the close work, and neck is more weary. But I'll not get teary!

BEN: Do you feel some verse coming on?

ME: No. Not today. But I've been singing this funny song, when I watch the workmen working in their trenches. It's about a hole in the ground. I only know the odd line and would love to sing the whole song. Could you find me the lyrics on the internet? I think it was sung by Bernard Cribbins.

BEN: Yep. Do you want to entertain the troops in their trenches?

ME: I might!


## Thursday 7th

8.42 a.m.

ME: After all the storms in the night, with wild winds – gale force something, the garden looks a *complete wreck*. Dustbin lids, neighbour's washing and bits of rubbish – not sure what – all over the lawn.

BEN: Yeah (yawning).

ME: Can you help me clear it up later?

BEN: Certainly dear.

\* \* \* \* \* \* \* \*

9.16 a.m. Ben helps me clear up the debris in the garden.

ME: Did you hear about the explosion in the cheese factory?

BEN: No.

ME: Dere was de Brie everywhere.

10.03 a.m.

ME: I've just been reading in Celebrity Weekly, Ronan Keating's wife's name is Storm. That's an unusual name. I imagine she was born on a night like last night. What do you think?

BEN: I'm sure you're right dear.

ME: I wonder if she has a frown like thunder clouds gathering, and her blue eyes flash like lightning when she's angry. She looks all joyful smiles in the photo of her with her baby bump, cuddling up to Ronan. Look, isn't it a sweet photo. I like her fluffy, pale grey jumper. She looks like a little cloud.

BEN: Very nice.

ME: They're not revealing the baby girl's name yet. I think they should call her Rain or Rainella, or Umberellie – Rellie for short.

BEN: Hailey, or Showerie.

ME: Or Cloudia. Storm says it will not be a traditional name, it'll be something a bit different. I can't wait to find out.

BEN: I expect other readers of Celebrity Weekly feel the same. Helps to sell copies. But most importantly, it'll be something for you to look forward to.

ME: When the baby is born and constantly wetting her nappies, they may decide to call her Puddle. And if she's like me, and grows up dyslexic with numbers and words, she'll be nicknamed Puddle in a muddle.

BEN: Now *I want* to know what they'll name her!

ME: I've got *Grand Designs* to look forward to tonight. Kevin McCloud follows a project to transform a nineteen-twenties cinema in Yorkshire, into a home.

BEN: Ronan Keating's surname should be McCloud.

ME: I quite agree. I can imagine Storm McCloud and baby Puddle splashing onto the next cover of Celebrity Weekly.

BEN: Celebrity Weekly love to *wet* the appetite of their readers!

11.36 a.m.

BEN: Steve is coming round tomorrow morning to help chop the bits off the hedge I can't reach, he's got the equipment for the job.

ME: Oh good, it has become a bit of an overgrown sight. It's grown so tall, it's as high as halfway up our bathroom window! Although I must admit, I enjoy the silhouette of the branches swaying in the wind, against the glowing light of an evening sunset when I'm in the bath. Don't you?

BEN: No, can't say I've noticed.

ME: Another thing I like, is where the hedge has grown so far across the garden, I can't see number eight's fence from the kitchen widow. But I do love to watch the shadows of the squirrels bounding along the fence, cast on the lawn when the sun comes round in the afternoon. I don't expect you've noticed them either.

BEN: Nope.

ME: Did you remember to ask Steve if he prefers cow's milk to soya milk in his tea or coffee?

BEN: I forgot. He may like almond milk!

ME: Somehow I doubt it. Oh, and we haven't got sugar, he may like sugar. It's so long since he last visited, I can't recall.

BEN: I'll ring 'im later.

\* \* \* \* \* \* \* \*

1.10 p.m.

BEN: Steve carries his own milk and sugar.

ME: Really!?

BEN:     His wife, Selena, runs her own gardening business and he helps out occasionally, and takes his provisions to their customers.

ME:     Ah, OK. I imagine that's a good idea if he's gardening for the elderly, or people like us who don't have sugar or cow's milk. Or maybe, because he's a gardener, people think he'll like a herb tea. And he's been so thirsty in the past, after working on a hot day, that he's had to endure a beverage that tastes like musty floorboards, old wardrobe or stale leaves.

BEN:     Eaten a lot of stale leaves, wardrobes and floorboards have we?

ME:     You know what I mean! But I do chew the carpet when you are hours late and I don't know where you are, and you're not answering your phone because you're in traffic. And I'm imagining all sorts of awful things!

BEN:     The front room carpet *is looking* a little frayed.

ME:     If Steve likes sugar, he probli likes a sweet treat and will like the milk chocolate Digestives you got for him.

BEN:     He might bring his own biscuits.

ME:     Yes. He may prefer a Garibaldi, a Bourbon, Custard Cream, shortbread, or just plain Digestives. No matter. We'll just have to eat 'em up.

BEN:     That will be awful.

ME:     Yes, terrible.

BEN: I remember the last time Bill came round to help with the decorating, you bought Digestives and a large pack of KitKats for him, and he said he's not keen on sweet things. So we had to eat them up – that was dreadful (smiling).

ME: Quite terrible.

BEN: Fortunately he loved the huge cheese and tomato rolls I made us.

ME: All this talk of biscuits is making me fancy a sweet treat. I must resist opening the choccy biccies. Once opened, we'll polish them off. Once bitten – want to bite again.

BEN: Think of musty floorboards and old wardrobes.

ME: I will......... It's not working....... Our old wardrobe is chocolate brown, and KitKats look like little floor boards you snap apart.

BEN: I'll print out the lyrics to that song you wanted – *Hole In The Ground*. You can have a nice sing, that'll work.

ME: Great! You can sing along with me.

BEN: Anything you say dear.

ME: *There I was, a-digging this hole*
*A hole in the ground, so big and sort of round it was*
*There was I, digging it deep*
*It was flat at the bottom and the sides were steep*
*When along comes this bloke in a bowler which he*
*lifted and scratched his head*

*Well he looked down the hole, the poor demented
soul and he said*

BEN: *Do you mind if I make a suggestion?*

ME: *Don't dig there, dig it elsewhere
You're digging it round and it ought to be square
The shape of it's wrong, it's much too long
And you can't put a hole where a hole don't belong*

BEN: *I ask you, what a liberty eh
Nearly bashed him right in the bowler*

ME: *Well there was I, stood in me hole
Shovelling earth for all I was worth
There was him, standing up there
So grand and official with his nose in the air
So I gave him a look sort of sideways and I leaned
on my shovel and sighed*

BEN: *Well I lit me a fag and having took a drag I replied*

ME: *I just couldn't bear, to dig it elsewhere
I'm digging it round cos I don't want it square
And if you disagree it doesn't bother me
That's the place where the hole's gonna be*

*Well there we were, discussing this hole
A hole in the ground so big and sort of round it was
Well it's not there now, the ground's all flat
And beneath it is the bloke in the bowler hat*

BEN: *And that's that.*

WE LAUGH

229

## Friday 8th

11.10 a.m.

BEN:    That's a sweet smile.

ME:    I've just enjoyed another choccy Digestive – pity Steve brought his Custard Creams. And he forgot to take the last of his packet home. SO thoughtless.

BEN:    Yeah (smiling and munching a Custard Cream).

ME:    But he lives about a forty-five minute journey away, so not much point in driving back, or you driving there for four biscuits.

BEN:    No (munch, munch).

ME:    It's not just the choccy treat making me smile. I'm re-lieved (perusing TV Weekly) I can watch *Coronation Street* tonight. I couldn't watch Monday's or Wednes-day's episodes because of the Shona and Clayton storyline. Either she'd be dead, or her son would be dead. Or they'd both be dead.

BEN:    Yeah (rolling eyes).

ME:    I saw that.

BEN:    With your wonderful peripheral vision.

ME:    Of course. Anyway, I got missing-*Coronation Street*-withdrawal-symptoms, and had to watch a repeat of Wednesday's episode. Shona and her son are still alive, David asked Shona to marry him, and Chesney has asked Gemma to move in with him (big sigh).

BEN: Great. So you're looking forward to tonight's episode.

ME: Yes (big smile), should be good. Lots of the characters are in a flap. Kevin, because Evelyn is missing. David and Nick, because of their new business. And Carla, because the Underworld's roof is leaking.

BEN: Well, I'm happy it will be most entertaining for you. Steve did a really good job on the hedge and wouldn't take any money, so I'm taking him out for a meal.

ME: Oh that's nice of him. Will you go for an Indian?

BEN: Yeah.

ME: Don't have one too hot, you know what happened last time you had a *really hot Indian!*

BEN: Yeah (pulling a face).

ME: Best avoid the Vindaloo. Korma is mild, but a bit too sweet and coconuty for you. What's the one you like? Vegetable Damask, or something?

BEN: Vegetable Dhansak. It's medium hotness.

ME: But if you go to the Tandoor Mahal, the chef there makes it fairly hot, so best have the yoghurty side dish to go with it – cucumber Rita or something.

BEN: Cucumber Raita dear..... I'm off in a minute to get loppers.

ME: You're off to get leopards? Did you and Steve make a pen to keep wild cats in, after you'd cut the hedge?

BEN: A lopper – it's like secateurs a with long handle.

ME: What are they for?

BEN: To chop up the large twigs from the hedge. Steve had one.

ME: Ah, good idea. Don't forget to get a birthday card for Paul – brother-in-law Paul. It's his birthday on Sunday so we need to send it first class today. I would have reminded you before today, but my leaky cauldron brain is getting leakier. Things I have to remember keep seeping out. Sweet treats are a good sealant.

BEN: I'm sure they are dear. I'll chop up the twigs and take them to the dump before it rains, then post Paul's card before the last post at four o'clock.

ME: Lovely. Two *round-twigs* – I mean *round-tuits* in one day!

\* \* \* \* \* \* \* \*

12.35 p.m.

BEN: Here you are, three cards.

ME: Three?...... Oh, they're really nice. You're so good at choosing cards. Who shall I write them to?

BEN: Paul's is the only urgent one.

ME: I'll write it *right away*. I take it Paul's is the one with the amusing drawings of bottles of beer.

BEN: Yeah. The one with the flowers and butterflies –

ME: And writing that looks like embroidery – sort of Jane Austen-ish...... Let me guess, your sister?

BEN: Julia, yeah.

ME: It's beautifully illustrated with delicate pastel colours – she'll love it.

BEN: The one with the dog is for Rob. Read what it says.

ME: OK..... *I was in a card shop today and found the FUNNIEST CARD I've ever seen! But it was nearly a fiver so I got this one. It has a doggy on it......* It's a perfect card. Will make him laugh.

BEN: And he loves his dog, Molly.

## Saturday 9th

10.00 a.m.

BEN: Did I hear a little cackle?

ME: It's just the title of this programme (nose in TV Week-ly), *The Dog Ate My Homework*. When I was twelve I had a friend whose parents had lots of little dogs running around their house. I can't recall how many or what breed, but I remember their house was very smelly! Anyway, my friend couldn't hand her home-work in one time, and she confided in me that one of the dogs *really had* chewed it up. Bless her.

11.30 a.m.

BEN:     Nice to hear you having another little cackle.

ME:      I'm watching *60 minute Makeover*. I'm enjoying all the flapping and flipping. Flapping of stripped off wallpaper, and flipping of tatty old brown sofa into a skip.

BEN:     Flopping of tired decorators in white dungarees at half-time.

* * * * * * * *

ME:      Flapping of ripped up drab carpet and flipping of new retro carpet into corners.

BEN:     Flopping of funky cushions onto stylish new sofa.

ME:      Flapping of funky dog silhouette wallpaper onto walls. Good paper isn't it!

BEN:     I expect you'd like the same, but with cats.

ME:      Yes! It would make a good feature wall in the back room......... I enjoy the last minute flapping at the end of the programme when it gets a bit chaotic. Arranging of cushions, ornaments and plants.

BEN:     Straightening of photos of dogs on the wall.

* * * * * * * *

ME:      That's really sweet!

BEN:     What is?

234

ME: Didn't you see? Freda and Keith's sheepdog barked with approval, and madly wagged its tail when they asked him what he thought of the makeover.

BEN: I was reading messages on my phone.

ME: You missed the best bit!

BEN: I'm sure I'll get over it in time.

12.05 p.m.

ME: What's that strange banging noise outside?

BEN: I can't hear anything.

ME: There it is again! There's bound to be windy-day-noises on a very windy March day, but this is right outside the back door.

BEN: Oh yeah! I can hear it now.... I'll investigate.

\* \* \* \* \* \* \* \*

BEN: The top part of the fence, near the back door, has broken away from the post.

ME: Don't leave it too long to sort it because like the hedge, it could become a bigger problem. It's stopped raining so now's your chance!

BEN: Don't fret dear, I'll get a *round-tuit* right away.

ME: Jane Austen would tell you to *make haste, make haste*, before we have most disagreeable weather.

12.15 p.m.

BEN: I've sorted the fence with a length of heavy duty, green earthing cable. It'll do for now. I'll get a metal angle bracket.

ME: You've done a grand job (peering out of the back door), I've never seen you get a *round-tuit* so quickly!

12.25 p.m.

ME: I must get a *round-tuit* myself in a minute.

BEN: What are you up to?

ME: Well, you know I've got a flour sieve sitting in the hedge, tied to the branches for the tiny birds to feed from?

BEN: Yeah, because the bigger birds and squirrels quickly devour the food on the bird table.

ME: But the big birds can't fly into the hedge and the squirrels *can* get in there but prefer the table.

BEN: Yeah, I know what you are going to say. Now the hedge has been trimmed back, the sieve feeder is more exposed and the bigger birds are eating the food for the little birds.

ME: Yes. Not the pigeons, but the collared doves and a pair of jays are. I'm going to put another slightly smaller sieve I've found, further in among the branches. I'll leave the other one where it is for now, in case it takes a while for the little birds to notice the new location. I'm going to use my Gardener's Mate.

BEN: Gardener's mate?

ME: You got it for me a while ago. It's like green, rubber pipe cleaner on a spool – called Twisty Tie. It's so easy to bend, I want to make little green animals out of it.

BEN: I'm surprised you haven't already dear.

ME: Anyway, the squirrels used to gnaw through string and take the sieve away, like a little basket of nuts. But they leave the Twisty Tie.

12.47 p.m.

ME: There's nothing like getting a *round-tuit* to make you feel better is there.

BEN: Absolutely.

ME: The blue tits have spotted their new feeder already!

BEN: Great. That's two more round tits – I mean *round-tuits* today. Well done us both!

ME: Yes. It must have been sad for the wee birdies to come down to breakfast and find just peanut husks left in the bottom of the sieve. Like you or I getting up to find just a few crumbs left in the bread bin, no bread in the freezer, and we've run out of tea, coffee and soya milk, and not even one water biscuit, Custard Cream or Digestive biscuit to share between us.

BEN: I quite agree dear.

3.11 p.m.

BEN:     What are you up to now?

ME:      You know you get those entertainers who make sausage dogs out of balloons?

BEN:     Yeah.

ME:      I'm making a little green dragon out of Twisty Tie.

BEN:     Are you going to twist again like you did last summer?

ME:      I am! I've made three loops and hung them on the kitchen cupboard door handles. Then found a red, yellow, and a green pepper with a very curly stalk and hung them on the hoops. Now the kitchen is wearing her best earrings – Look!

BEN:     Very nice dear.

ME:      *Come on let's twist again*
         *Like we did last summer!*
         *Yeaah, lets twist again*
         *Like we did last year!*

BEN:     *Do you remember when*
         *Things were really hummin'*
         *Yeaah, lets twist again*
         *Twistin' time is here!*

WE LAUGH

5.26 p.m.

BEN:    I fancy pancakes again tonight.

ME:     Why not! Have we got all the ingredients (talking to self).... Erm...... *think*...... *think*...... got flour, lemon juice, salt....... milk and honey..... Do you know I've sometimes wondered why a honeymoon is called a honeymoon, and now I know why.

BEN:    I can't wait to be enlightened.

ME:     I read yesterday in Weekly Wife, that for a month after a Babylonian wedding, the bride's father-in-law would supply his son-in-law with all the mead, or honey beer, he could drink. This was known as the honey month. Now the honeymoon!

BEN:    Fascinating..... We need eggs too.

ME:     Oh yes.


## Sunday 10th

10.10 a.m.

ME:     Nice sunny day for Paul's birthday. And travelling. Is your nephew still picking you up, then your great niece, and taking you both to Paul and Julia's?

BEN:    We've had to change our plans.

ME:     Oh, why?

BEN:    Strong winds have disrupted things, it's a long story

ME: Is it long-*winded*?

BEN: I'm afraid so.

ME: Goody, *love* a long story. But of course I'm sorry to know things aren't going to plan.

BEN: Are you sitting comfortably?

ME: Yes, very.

BEN: Then I'll begin. At the Dartford Tunnel there is now also a very high suspension bridge called the QE2 Bridge. The old tunnel works in conjunction with the new bridge, so these days both 'bores' of the tunnel take the traffic from Kent to Essex, whereas before the bridge was built, one bore went Kent to Essex and the other bore, Essex to Kent...... pretty *boring* so far!

ME: No, no. Do continue.

BEN: These days the whole shebang is called the Dartford Crossing. However, when the winds are very strong they have to close the bridge because it can become unsafe, particularly for taller vehicles like lorries and buses...... which incidentally was exactly what those opposed to the bridge said would happen! And they also suggested another tunnel should be built instead.

ME: Oh dear. Some people don't listen to sense do they.

BEN: When the bridge is closed they revert to having the two halves of the tunnel only, with one half going Kent to Essex and the other half going Essex to Kent. Because there is so much more traffic than there used to be, everything on both sides of the crossing gets very slow and congested.

ME:        I can imagine.

BEN:      So we knew we'd have to delay getting across the Thames...... but then the icing on the cake was that Kira's train from Canterbury to Maidstone East was cancelled due to the high winds that had apparently brought the power lines down. She had walked all the way to Canterbury station before she found out, it's a long walk too.

ME:        Poor Kira!

BEN:      The plan was for my nephew to drive over, pick me up, then pick Kira up from Maidstone East, then head for Paul and Julia's house and hope we could dodge as much traffic as possible using our 'local knowledge'. Now we are driving to Canterbury first, to pick up Kira, but hopefully we'll get to our destination on time.

ME:        And all live happily ever after..... The End.

* * * * * * * *

*You do not find the happy life. You make it.*

Camilla Eyring Kimball

**Five and a bit months later**

# September

**Sunday 1st**

10.02 a.m.  I sleepily watched a tiny, fluffy white feather float dreamily down from the heavenly blue September sky – as if falling from the warm wing of a passing angel. A white butterfly appeared from out of the blue and fluttered around it. They danced together for a while to the rhythm of the cool morning breeze – Mother Nature's waltz. Then disappeared from view like lovers deeply in love, wanting to be alone together, and gaze lovingly into each other's eyes. And kiss with gentle butterfly kisses. Forever.

10.03 a.m.  While I waited for the kettle to boil, I sang a few lines of song by ABBA, changing some of the words.

*I believe in angels*
*Something good in everything I see*

*I see angel feathers*
*Dancing with the butterflies and bees*
*Under the trees*
*September breeze*

Then I drifted into the garden wearing my floaty, white dressing gown, to give the birds a late morning treat. Moments later a tiny, grey feather rested in the palm of my hand, as the collared doves descended. I smiled at their bright little eyes, and the single rose, still blooming and pink as my cheeks from the warm kitchen – gently nodding with approval of feathers dancing with butterflies, soft grey doves, and the blooming beautiful day. A tiny sycamore seed, caught in a spider's web, twirled like a flamenco dancer wearing a frilly, satin, red dress, and I felt inspired to burst into song again. A song I knew very few words to.

*I love it when you call me senorita*
*I wish I could pretend I didn't need ya*

*Be do, be do, be do, la la la*
*It's true, la, la, la*

10.14 a.m.

BEN: You sound very cheerful!

ME: I am. Now the weather is cooler and I can sleep better, and it's all quiet on the building site front today. That was one hell of a heatwave.

BEN: Hot as hell.

ME: Today is heavenly. Angels fill the sky.

BEN: Have you been cloud watching again dear?

ME: I've been feather watching.

BEN: Nice to have a new hobby.

ME: You'll be flying soon, on your mini-break. Send me lots of lovely messages so I feel I'm there too.

BEN: Will do.

ME: I expect it'll be blissfully quiet where you'll be staying, and you'll have a beautiful break from the constant noise here.

BEN: Looking forward to it!

ME: I'm making the most of the peace today. The workmen will be at home, looking forward to Sunday dinner with their family, then snoozing in front of the TV, watching *Stewart Little 2* on ITV.

BEN: Or down the pub with their mates.

ME: Or enjoying a romantic almost-Autumn stroll with their girlfriends......... And talking of romance, I'm *most* looking forward to Jane Austen's *Sanditon* this afternoon. Charlotte and Sidney clash again, Esher and Edward realise that Clara poses a threat to their ambitions, while tensions surrounding Miss Lambe erupt at Lady Denham's grand luncheon.

BEN: That all sounds *most agreeable* m'lady.

## Monday 2nd

8.12 a.m.

BEN: What's making you cackle my little witch?

ME: The titles of some of these programmes – *Bangers and Cash,* about cars in an auction.

BEN: Do you fancy veggie bangers and mash for dinner?

ME: Sounds tasty.

BEN: Peas and gravy?

ME: Lovely!....... We've almost run out of gravy granules,

I must put them on your shopping list before you go away.

BEN:    OK.

ME:     *Junk and Disorderly* is a good title, about motorcycle memorabilia...... No, no, I'm not going to say it reminds me of you after a Friday night out with your mates!

BEN:    *Junk and Disorderly* sounds like our cellar.

ME:     Yes. Even though we've de-cellared........ no....... defrosted.... no.... can't think of the word.

BEN:    De-cluttered?

ME:     Ah, thank you. You're always finding the words I lose!....... *Bin There, Dump That* – that's another good one....... Don't forget to put the rubbish out tonight. I've stuffed all the wrapping from your *round-tuits* in a bin bag. It's in the back room, so don't forget that either.

BEN:    No dear.

ME:     There's a programme on today – *Food Unwrapped*. The presenter visits McVitie's in Carlisle to find out why so many biscuits are covered in holes.

BEN:    You know what will happen if you watch that.

ME:     Yes dear (licking lips, a glacé cherry glint in my eye).

* * * * * * * *

8.35 a.m.

BEN:       What's making you sad my little witch?

ME:         I'm alright. It's just the racket has started up on the building site and I've got the back-to-all-the-noise-Monday-morning-blues. Back to the relentless hammering and sound of nail guns banging away – our own little war zone. How nice.

BEN:       Yeah.

ME:         Then there's the sound like a giant hoover, making dogs bark and babies cry lots of tears. Cats frown and flatten their ears. And it feels like it'll go on for years.

BEN:       Birds complain on Twitter.

ME:         Breeze blows the litter.

BEN:       Beer tastes too bitter.

ME:         Do we feel a poem coming on?

BEN:       No. Not today.

ME:         At least, now the weather is cooler and Autumn is on its way, we can shut the windows. And this time next year –

BEN:       We'll be millionaires!

ME:         I doubt it, Derek Trotter (giggling). The building work will be completed and people will be viewing the flats and houses.

BEN:    And if you get to speak to one of the young couples, you will say, pointing to the flats, 'This was an orchard once upon a time, that's why we are Orchard Street.' Then you'll point to where the tarmac doesn't quite cover the cobbles near the path and say, 'And our little street was cobbled, like in *Coronation Street*'. Then you'll show them our apple green door, in memory of the orchard.

ME:    And they'll smile at the strange little *Coronation Street* loving old lady, and pretend to admire our newly painted, glossy green door, with glossy black knocker, and to be most enthralled by my wonderful piece of information about the orchard and cobbles. And when they move in we will wave to them across the street, and they'll wave back. And we'll take in parcels for them like we do for number 6 and number 8. And we'll all live happily ever after.

BEN:    You and your happy endings!

5.23 p.m.

ME:    Oh dear.

BEN:    What's up?

ME:    I've started a shopping list for you, before you go away. Did you notice the photo on the calendar in the kitchen for this month?

BEN:    I did. A slice of chocolate gateau.

ME:    Topped with tasty looking choccy swirls and raspberries.

BEN: And you need comfort food when I'm away, so top of the list is –

ME: Yes...... Wendy of Weekly Wife tells me, with the changeable weather approaching, it makes sense to layer your clothes. But I'd rather be eating three layers –

BEN: Of choccy sponge?

ME: Correct (giggling). And I shouldn't have watched *Food Unwrapped.*

BEN: So now McVitie's choccy Digestive biccies are next on the list?

ME: Mm. And I'm tempted to add Jaffa Cakes and Nice biccies... they are *so nice!*.... Can't help it! I always want to comfort eat when you're away. I don't know what happened to my healthy M.E. diet. I think aliens landed and took it away from me. Yes...... Yes...... I'll blame the aliens. They beamed me up from our street, into their spaceship and took me to the planet SUGAR. A wonderful place, where sugary foods are very good for your health. The more cake and biscuits and chocolate and ice cream you eat, the better you feel, and the slimmer you get. *And* you have *so much energy!*..... And everyone smiles all day. And everything you experience in life is sugar coated, so tastes sweeter. And there's no pollution because everyone rides on sparkly white unicorns, and everyone has sparkly white teeth, so they never need to go to the dentist.

BEN: I understand dear, the lack of my wonderful company must be most distressing for you.

ME: I've been good all summer, eating lots of healthy salads, well most of the summer, so I deserve a treat.

*Honey, la, la, la, la, la, la*
*Ah, sugar, sugar*

BEN: *You are my candy girl*
*And you got me wanting you!*

WE LAUGH

## Tuesday 3rd

9.20 a.m.

ME: I'm *so glad* you're not flying off till tomorrow. I'd not have been able to carry the heavy rubbish bags and food bin from the back yard to the front of the house today. I count my blessings I have a big strong man.

BEN: Good to be appreciated!

\* \* \* \* \* \* \* \*

11.25 a.m. Ben plods in through the front door laden with two yellow (with an orange elephant on the side) Sainsbury's carrier bags, with the slogan – strong and sturdy.

ME: I'm so fortunate I have a strong and sturdy man to do shopping and carry heavy things.

BEN: Great (laughing). Tell me what you want opening before I go.

ME: Will do. Jar of mayonnaise and bottles of water for a start. I'm so lucky to have a strong, sturdy man to carry things, open things, squidge things out of tubes, find words when I lose them and *catch spiders*. Please don't die in a plane crash!

BEN: Is there a spider needs catching?

ME: Yes. It's a huge monster! Wendy of Weekly Wife said an explosion of spider sightings is due mid-September, as the weather cools. And there's a spider catcher you can get now, from ALDI. It looks good – like a plastic pyramid on the end of a stick. You put the pyramid over the spider, then there's a slidey bit that traps it, so you can take it outside, un-slide the slidey bit and set it free. Can you get one when you get back from your trip?

BEN: Yep. We don't want spiders exploding all over the house do we dear.

\* \* \* \* \* \* \* \* \*

11.27 a.m. I'm helping Ben put the shopping away. Diamanda watches, whiskers twitching, as she counts the number of cans of tuna being placed in the cupboard. She likes to have plenty in stock.

11.28 a.m. As I pick up the light things (teabags, Digestives, Jaffa Cakes, toilet roll), I watch Ben place a can of beans next to the tuna.

ME: I've never seen those beans before, Prosecco beans?!

BEN: Rosecoco beans.

ME:      Oh, you usually only get Heinz baked beans, and butter beans to make your veggie burgers.

BEN:      I thought I'd like to try them for a change.

ME:      The label says they help you create authentic Asian cuisine, wherever you are in the world.

BEN:      Great, I'll use them in one of my curries!

ME:      Wendy of Weekly Wife also informed me, Heinz is celebrating its one hundred and fiftieth year, and there was a temporary museum honouring its baked beans.

BEN:      That's nice (placing a can of Heinz beans next to a jar of Hellmann's mayonnaise).

ME:      The UK consumes over five hundred and fifty *million* cans of beans a year (opening the Jaffa Cakes).

BEN:      Fascinating. The population must be full of beans (placing the frozen chips in the freezer).

ME:      Diamanda is very full of beans these days.

BEN:      At the moment she is *fish-full* thinking.

ME:      That she is! I'll open a nice fresh can for her, I'm getting the spooky *feed-me-now* stare.

BEN:      It'll never be as spooky as your cat painting, now it's finished.

ME:      That's true. Would you like a Jaffa Cake or two with your coffee?

BEN:       Yeah!

ME:        Jaffa Cakes are like cats. It's hard to have just one.

* * * * * * * *

4.10 p.m.

ME:        Peace at last. You must be *SO looking forward* to getting away, after an extra noisy building site day.

BEN:       Yeah!

ME:        There's a lot of programmes on at the moment about flying. *The Secret Life of the Long-Haul Flight, Flights From Hell: Caught On Camera* and *Flights from Hell: Terror in The Skies*. It's making me nervous about tomorrow. Who are you flying with?

BEN:       My sister.

ME:        Very funny.

BEN:       We're flying with Ryanair.

ME:        I need comfort food tonight.

BEN:       Burgers, Heinz beans and oven chips?

ME:        Perfect.

## Wednesday 4th

12.34 p.m.   As a big lorry rumbles by, the house shakes, and I can't shake off an uneasy feeling about Ben's flight. I love to fly, and love to fly with Ben, and *never* get nervous – I can't wait to get on the plane and be above the white clouds. It's heavenly. But today I feel different. I have a *gloomy grey **feeling*** that all is not well. And I can't wait for him to be back home, safe and sound. I think I may have to eat ***all*** the contents of the fridge, freezer and kitchen cupboards.

1.25 p.m.   I shouldn't have polished off the Jaffa Cakes after the hearty vegetable soup and a sandwich.

2.20 p.m.   Ben sends a text message:

ARRIVED AT STANSTED AIRPORT – LOOKS LIKE FLIGHT MAY BE DELAYED

2.21 p.m.   I reply:

OH, THAT-S A PAIN – AT LEAST YOU HAVE GOOD COMPANY

2.22 p.m.   YES, WE ARE HAVING A GIGGLE

2.23 p.m.   BON VOYAGE XX

2.24 p.m.   I wonder if the plane is delayed due to terrible weather conditions. Or one of the wheels dropped off and they had to stick it back on again...... When they finally take-off they may run into severe storms, suffer lots of turbulence, fly off-course and crash into the French Alps.

2.25 p.m.   I crack open the McVitie's chocolate digestives.

3.23 p.m.   I'm sitting in the garden. Warm sun on my face. Chocolate on my lips. Diamanda, Celebrity Weekly and TV Weekly for company.

3.24 p.m.    I gaze up into the sky and watch a plane make white tracks across the soft, September blue. I give the plane a little wave, Ben may be on that flight on his way to France.

3.25 p.m.    The sky becomes sad September blues. I may never, *ever* see him again.

3.26 p.m.    Then I smile, remembering Ben bought Camembert, French bread, and a bottle of wine – Bordeaux (opened and breathing nicely), to help me visualise being with him in the suburbs of Bordeaux..... If he gets there safely.

3.27 p.m.    The word Bordeaux makes me think of gateau.

3.28 p.m.    I must not think of gateau yet, have had two choccy biccies and *too many* Jaffa Cakes.

3.30 p.m.    I plod, feeling ten pounds heavier, indoors to the kitchen.

3.34 p.m.    Mmmm....... Gateau is so inspiring. Makes me think of the word chateau. And the lovely French chateau being renovated by Dick and Angel, in *Escape To The Chateau.* Maybe I'll write some verse about eating gateau and sipping Cointreau, while lounging on an art nouveau chaise longue, admiring a pain-painting by Henry Rousseau at a chateau in Bordeaux.

3.36 p.m.    Do I feel inspired to write poetry? I duneau.

\* \* \* \* \* \* \* \* \*

3.48 p.m.    Back in the garden, Celebrity Weekly tells me it's a good time to fly to Cyprus. The summer hordes will be gone, it's an ideal place for autumnal sunshine, and less than a four hour flight from the UK.

I wonder how long it will take Ben to get to his destination, can't wait to hear he's safely tucked up in his B&B in Bordeaux.

3.49 p.m.   I enjoy perusing photos of turquoise waters, a deserted coastline at Paphos, picturesque cobbled streets, white-washed stone houses and beautiful ancient architecture. But feel happy in my little garden, enjoying the many shades of green, sitting on my ancient garden bench, my broomstick leaning against the white-washed wall (it's about time it had another MOT) and the workmen in our nail-gun-banging little war zone have ceased fire for the day. Peace at last.

3.52 p.m.   Turning the pages, past *Emmerdale's* stars Charley and Matthew welcoming their third son (I never watch the programme so I'm not interested) and Simon Cowell's views (can't stand the man) and radio presenter Ashley Roberts talks about feeling broody (never heard of her), I see a familiar face smiling out of the pages at me – *Grand Designs* presenter Kevin McCloud. He is going to be celebrating the show's 20th anniversary, with a selection of some of his favourite chocolates (I mean projects) in a special episode entitled, *Kevin's Grand Designs*.

3.53 p.m.   I wonder if he has favourite chocolates. Maybe like me, he loves perfect little leaf-shaped mint chocolates – plain, milk and white. He enjoys perfection. Thorntons do some grand designs with their confectionary – artistically arranged in boxes with red ribbon and a bow for the finishing touch. He likes an attractive finishing touch. And also appreciates hand craftsmanship, so he may enjoy handmade truffles, like the ones Ben hand-picked for me once from a little shop near Camden Lock, with a lovely selection of flavours – hazelnut praline, Belgian dark chocolate, vanilla, spiced biscuit and espresso coffee.

3.56 p.m.    Sipping coffee with a choccy biccie and more of the interview with Kevin in Celebrity Weekly. His answer to one of the questions made me cackle quite loudly, and I wished Ben was home to hear me. My cackles make him smile. I hope he's having a good flight.

Kevin was asked if there were any common traits in a Grand Designer. He said there was a sort of glint in the eye, a sort of self-righteousness that meant whatever he told them they were going to ignore. The fact that he's seen hundreds of projects and has made observations about all of them is of no relevance to most of the self-builders he has met, who are just absolutely convinced that their project is going to be the one that goes right. Then he adds a BUT..... But where this springs from is hope – the wonderful, human fallibility that we all have, which is hope.

I REALLY HOPE Ben and his sister have landed, or soon will land safely in France.

4.04 p.m.    Ben sends a text:

FLIGHT NOW WON-T LEAVE TILL 20 TO 7 – SO RYANAIR ARE OFF MY XMAS CARD LIST

4.05 p.m.    I reply:

OH, SORRY TO HEAR THAT – YOU AND JULIA SHOULD

TREAT YOURSELVES TO A TASTY SNACK BEFORE YOUR
FLIGHT X

4.07 p.m.     Ben replied:

WE WILL X

4.10 p.m.     I sit.

4.11 p.m.     I sip a calming camomile tea.

4.12 p.m.     Wearing a worried face.

I wonder if the delay is a technical problem. Is the
old plane starting to fall apart. Is there a problem
with the engine? Is the door not closing properly? It
can only take a minor fault to cause a big problem –
I've watched programmes about it. A bit like the
human body sometimes – suddenly you feel so fatigued you fly off the handle, in the wrong direction.
And you are not sure why.

4.15 p.m.     I feel the need to text Ben:

DO YOU KNOW WHAT IS CAUSING THE DELAY?

4.20 p.m.     He hasn't replied yet.

4.21 p.m.     I wish he'd reply.

4.22 p.m.     Must stay calm.

4.23 p.m.     Pick up phone to send him another message, but
just as I begin to do this a message comes through
– hurrah!

It's just my phone people telling me they've topped up my account.

4.25 p.m.    Another text!...... It's just my brother saying hello and telling me his news. Will reply a bit later.

I need a drink of the nicely breathing wine..... but not a good idea, it'll make me too emotional. If I get bad news I will be a mess.

4.29 p.m.    Ooh, another text, mustn't get too excited, may not be Ben:

THE FLIGHT TO HERE FROM BORDEAUX HASN-T ARRIVED YET, SO SOMETHING MUST HAVE DELAYED TAKE OFF AT BORDEAUX

4.30 p.m.    I replied, resisting the urge to ask why he had taken so long to reply to my last message, and not telling him I had a bad feeling, because he knows my bad feelings often come true, and now I'm wondering if there is a bomb scare or something, and I want him and his sister to come home now. PLEASE!

Decide to watch Tony Robinson on *Time Team* to calm me down.

4.31 p.m.    I see in TV Weekly, it's a repeat. The one where they're not searching for ancient Roman ruins or a nice medieval castle. They are in the middle of a field, digging up the remains of a World War Two plane crash. I don't believe it!

4.32 p.m.    I'll watch *Friends* on Channel 5.

It's the one where Rachel is on a plane. She is flying

to England to see Ross, who is about to marry Emily, but she needs to tell him she loves him. It's a very funny episode, especially as Hugh Laurie is in it and he is SO hilarious. But I can't watch it. Will watch *Most Haunted* at 5.00 p.m.

5.10 p.m.　Yvette and her team of ghost hunters are not in a lovely old haunted castle or mansion, or a creepy old pub with glasses flying about at night, and evil smugglers whispering in their ears. Drat. They are in a World War Two aircraft carrier, and the guest medium is feeling a burning sensation on his arms.

5.11 p.m.　I give up watching TV. Turn the radio on. Elton John is singing, 'Daniel is flying tonight on a plane'.

5.15 p.m.　I sit. Staring out of the bedroom window at a wall of bricks, with gaps ready for the window panes. I don't care that my view has gone, just want Ben and his sister to come home safely.

5.40 p.m.　Thinking about preparing veg for dinner.

5.44 p.m.　Don't think I can eat anything. Just fancy a glass of wine.

5.45 p.m.　Can't eat or relax with a glass of wine until I know Ben and his sister are safely in France, nice and cosy in their B&B.

6.00 p.m.　In bathroom. One green toothbrush in the holder looks lonely. She feels blue.

6.01 p.m.　I hope their (I mean there) will soon be two toothbrushes together again.

6.50 p.m.    My tummy rumbles.

6.51 p.m.    I nibble a small slice of French bread, not really tasting it. I'm watching *Poirot*. Haven't a clue what's going on, but am relieved it's not the episode where he's on a plane most of the time.

7.15 p.m.    I had planned to watch my favourite episode of *Absolutely Fabulous* (the one where Patsy and Edina travel to France, and sample too much wine at a chateau) with a glass of Bordeaux, French bread and French cheese (me eating the French bread and cheese, not Patsy and Edina). But there are scenes where they are on a plane, and at the end, at customs. Will watch *Coronation Street* at 7.30. I will find out if Eileen has departed with Jan, and if Sean finds out about Eileen's plans and tries to stop her. That will take my mind off things.

8.00 p.m.    *Heathrow: Britain's Busiest Airport* is on. Change channel to watch Kevin McCloud in *Grand Designs*. Tonight he is on a clifftop in Scotland.

8.30 p.m.    Part two of *Coronation Street*.

8.33 p.m.    Ooh, a text message!

    LANDED X

8.34 p.m.    I reply:

    THAT-S ABSOLUTELY FABULOUS !!

8.35 p.m.    I pour a glass of wine, and plan to enjoy lots of warmed French bread, spread with Camembert, with my favourite episode of *Absolutely Fabulous,* after

*Coronation Street.*

9.12 p.m.   Patsy and Edina are getting very merry in the wine cellar of a chateau. I laugh along with them, but still have a bit of an uneasy feeling.

9.33 p.m.   Ben sends another text:

JUST TO PUT THE KYBOSH ON THE TRAVELLING DAY – WE ARE STUCK WAITING TO GO THRU CUSTOMS TO MAIN AIRPORT CUZ OF A SECURITY SCARE – THEY DON-T KNOW HOW LONG FOR  - BUT WE ARE SAFE X

9.34 p.m.   I reply:

OH WHAT A PAIN – YOU AND JULIA MUST BE EXHAUSTED – STAY SAFE XX

9.35 p.m.   They may not be safe really. *Is this really happening?*

9.36 p.m.   I pour another glass of wine. But don't drink it.

* * * * * * * *

10.12 p.m.   Another text from Ben:

IN CAB – ON WAY TO B & B X

10.13 p.m.   I replied, then sighed a *huge sigh* and plodded off to bed.

## Thursday 5th

9.01 a.m.   I watch the rain drizzling down the window pane.

Drilling down... down... down into the lawn.

9.02 a.m.    Down onto the leaves of our hedge. They look like they are waving goodbye to the summer.

I see my first autumn leaves of the year fall down.... down.... down.... from our sycamore tree into long blades of grass.

9.03 a.m.    I try not to feel down, after nightmares about a bomb exploding on a plane, then it crashes into the Eiffel Tower.

9.05 a.m.    I pop a camomile teabag into a mug and pour water from the kettle down over it.

9.06 a.m.    I feel the need to pour my feelings out to someone. Maybe I'll write them down.

9.35 a.m.    Rain continues to fall.
Down... down... down.... down... down.

9.36 a.m.    I try not to feel down as I recall my nightmare again. When the plane exploded little bodies fell from the sky, like those matchstick people painted by the English painter who painted industrial landscapes. Can't recall his name. Something beginning with **L**... Lawrence?... Larry?... Laurie?

9.38 a.m.    Can't help feeling low. I'll be OK when Ben is home safe and sound. Hope he's having a good time. I'll cheer up when I hear from him.

9.40 a.m.    Feel low... low... low... Lowry! L. S. Lowry. That was his name!

9.51 a.m.    Received a cheerful text from Ben:

GREAT WEATHER – LOOKING FORWARD TO DAY OUT – DAVE ARRIVED FROM BARCELONA LAST NIGHT AFTER FLIGHT DELAYS – ARRIVED BEFORE US SO DID SHOPPING AND COOKED FOR US X

I replied, feeling uplifted:

THAT-S LOVELY – HAVE A GOOD DAY OUT – LOOK FORWARD TO HEARING FROM YOU LATER X

9.52 a.m.    I felt relieved that Ben's brother had arrived in France safely. I'd had not-so-good feelings about his flight too. Double-worry deserves double choc gateau. Will indulge while watching *Escape To The Chateau* at midday...... Mmm..... maybe just a small slice now.

11.10 a.m.    I sang as I did the washing-up. I know I'm OK if I'm singing.

*And he painted matchstalk men and matchstalk cats and dogs*

*He painted kids on the corner of –*

Diamanda padded into the kitchen, stopping me in mid-verse and demanded a tuna treat. I can tell she's missing Ben, she kept sitting by the front door last night. With droopy whiskers. Waiting.

11.11 a.m.    I gave her an extra big treat and lots of fuss.

11.21 a.m.    I picked up the washing-up brush and finished the washing-up.

*Now he takes his brush and he waits outside them factory gates*

*To paint his matchstalk men and matchstalk cats and dogs*

\* \* \* \* \* \* \* \*

12.45 p.m.  The September sun has appeared and is shining brightly between ash grey clouds. I'm sitting in the garden with Celebrity Weekly and Weekly Wife – the breeze turning the pages for me, never fails to amuse me. Especially on days when just turning a page feels like a humongous effort.

12.46 p.m.  A page in Weekly Wife is turned to a short story entitled, *One September In France,* by Katie Ashmore, with a very beautiful photo of golden and crimson autumn leaves. I admire the photo, then read the first few lines before the breeze turns the pages to the end of the magazine.

*John walked down the Rue Chanson and raised his jacket collar. It was a blustery September day. A thin sun poked its way between dove grey clouds; fallen leaves swirled at his feet.*

12.47 p.m.  Good start. I like the description of the clouds being dove grey. Will read the rest of the story later. I think I'll just sit and enjoy the wildlife for a while. The workmen on the building site are at lunch, so our world is peaceful.

12.48 p.m.  I watch a tiny snail slowly and slimily slither up the side of my garden bench. His delicate little horns swaying from side to side, as if he is thinking –

Which way now?... What direction should I take?... What shall I do next?..... A bit like Ben decorating our house – slowly getting there, but not sure what to tackle next. He points his horns at every new challenge. But sometimes. Quite often. Most of the time really these days, he will just retreat into his shell (put headphones on and listen to the music he is composing). But there's no hurry to decorate. And his music his is joyfully jazzy. *And* Diamanda thinks it's cool for cats. So do I. And we're not so bothered about moving urgently now anyway. We'll slither along in our own time. Our own rhythm of daily life. And wait to see what it's like living opposite the new housing estate next year.

12.49 p.m.    I sit. Very, very still. I'm playing statues. Just like the squirrels do on our our fence when they sense a big, hairy feline with lots of claws and teeth is nearby. I don't turn my head or make the slightest movement. Just blink. And slowly turn my eyes sideways to watch one of our squirrels spring sprightly onto the bird table next to me. I turn my head *very slowly*, very slightly, and delight in watching her stuff her little grey, whiskery face with as many peanuts as she can, till her cheeks bulge. Then she bounces away along the fence to find the next place to bury her stash – beautiful, bushy tail twitching.... little paws galloping at super-speed.... *hurry... hurry...* Autumn is on it's way... *boing!... boing!... boing!*

12.50 p.m.    I enjoy the memory of when I was on my way to work, back in the eighties. I'd walk through a small park. Brenchley Gardens. And feed the squirrels. They would clamber up my arms and over my shoulders... *boing!... boing!... boing!* It was one the sweetest, most lovely wildlife experiences I've ever

266

had. If I was a bit late for work sometimes at the drawing office in St. Peter's Street, everyone knew why – she's been with the squirrels again!

1.04 p.m.    A tiny money spider crawls across the fashion pages of Celebrity Weekly. A sultry model with perfectly tousled blonde hair, serene in a scarlet berry print dress, is leaning against an ivy covered stone wall. I smile as I imagine moments later she will be screaming with fright when a creepy-crawly creeps out of the ivy, over her shoulder and down her cleavage.

1.05 p.m.    The breeze turns the page. The same model, wearing a pretty, pink rose print dress, is sitting on a stone wall holding an armful of white roses. Her eyes look a little watery. Is it the chilly wind or has she just been stabbed in the arm by a sharp rose thorn?

1.07 p.m.    Perusing the travel pages, I wonder what Ben is doing. I long to hear from him, and feel a little stab of pain at the thought of him never coming home again.

1.09 p.m.    The recipe page looks mouth-watering – almost the whole page is a photo of an Italian salad. A simple salad. Just buffalo mozzarella, fresh tomatoes and basil, drizzled with olive oil, and sprinkled with salt and freshly ground pepper. But gazing at the photo I can *almost smell* the fresh basil and newly sliced tomatoes, the salt and ground pepper enhancing their taste, and want to get a knife and fork and get stuck in.

1.11 p.m.    As I make a sandwich filled with cottage cheese, slices of tomato, and sprinkled with ground black pepper, I hope Ben enjoyed a tasty French lunch in a nice little French café.

2.00 p.m.    I wonder where he is now.

2.01 p.m.    Hope he and his sister and brother are having a good time. After their very sad summer, they need a nice little break. Together.

2.02 p.m.    To take my mind off sad thoughts, I continue to read the short story in Weekly Wife.

*Pedestrians hurried to their destinations, their heads bent. John thrust his hands deeper into his pockets and strode on towards his apartment by the river. It had been a difficult day, but he was coping better, living here in France.*

2.03 p.m.    Is that my phone?!

2.04 p.m.    No. It's a pedestrian's phone, hurrying to their destination past our house, head bent and collar raised against the September breeze.

2.05 p.m.    I carry on reading.

*This morning at the garage where he worked, someone had dropped a spanner. The clang had resounded through the whole building.*

2.06 p.m.    There is a loud *CLANG* and a *CRASH* on the building site followed by lots of naughty words, followed by more relentless nail-gun-banging.

2.07 p.m.    I decide to retreat to the back room, close the door, put Ben's headphones on, and listen to his music. Then realise I will not hear the ringtone on my phone, so I sit the phone in front of me, where I can see when a message comes through.

2.12 p.m.     Diamanda appears and sits on my phone.

2.13 p.m.     As I heave my old human body out of the chair and head for the kitchen to give her a treat, she lifts her lovely feline body, in a gracious way, up to follow me. So I quickly go back to retrieve the phone, pop it in my cardie pocket, then give her a tuna treat. Gracious young cats are very good at training their old humans to give them a treat when they desire.

2.30 p.m.     Diamanda curls up for an afternoon sleep, so I sit the phone in front of me again. Am tempted to send Ben a text message.

* * * * * * * * *

3.20 p.m.     Was VERY tempted to text Ben. Hadn't heard from him for five hours, twenty-nine minutes and fifteen seconds.

3.21 p.m.     Was VERY tempted to devour all the contents of the fridge and cupboards for the next five hours, twenty-nine minutes and fifteen seconds.

3.23 p.m.     As I picked up my phone a text came through.

HAD A NICE FEW HOURS VISITING THE AMAZING CITY DU VIN WHICH IS A VERY ARTY MODERN BUILDING FULL OF WINE RELATED EXHIBITIONS – AND YOU GET A FREE GLASS OF WINE

3.24 p.m.     I giggled, knowing Ben only has to *look* at a glass of wine and he's tipsy. One glass and he's merry. So I replied:

I EXPECT YOU ARE A MERRY TOURIST NOW

He replied:

YES A BIT MERRY – WITH VERY TIRED FEET X

3.25 p.m.   I grinned, and thought I may have an early glass of
wine myself with a couple of slices of French bread,
spread with Camembert (cherry tomato on top –
a savoury version of an iced cupcake with a glacé
cherry on top), followed by gateau, all nicely digested
with a delicious episode of *Poirot*. Parfait.

## Friday 6th

10.20 a.m.   A flyer flew in through the letter box, advertising
Pilates classes in our town. I read it as Pilots classes.

10.21 a.m.   I stood by the front door, hoping that Ben's pilot for
his next flight was well trained for an emergency.

10.22 a.m.   I looked forward to Ben coming home tomorrow,
and hoped he wouldn't suffer more delays at the
airports.

10.23 a.m.   I thought pilots who have delayed flights should be
called Pilates.

11.04 a.m.   Sipping a minty tea, I felt relieved Ben would be
home soon, because Diamanda has started moping
around the house meowing, then curling up on his
pillow with sad-cat eyes. He'd sent a text earlier when
I was in the garden feeding the wildlife and talking

to a snail with very handsome horns. Today he (Ben not the snail, although I'm sure snails must have lots of lovely adventures) would be getting a tram, then taking a short boat trip to Bordeaux.

11.35 a.m.    Lots of lovely post arrived. Among the boring looking envelopes were colourful catalogues: Joe Browns, Culture Vulture, Natural Health Matters (end of summer sale) and Museum Selection. Promising nice little perusing sessions.

11.50 a.m.    With the weather turning chillier today, the cosy looking cable jumpers, cardies and hooded knits in Joe Browns looked lovely and warm and tempting to buy, *and* most appealing in shades of plum, teal, mustard, olive green and coffee.

11.52 a.m.    I sipped hot coffee. Not the de-caf I should be drinking. Ben's *real* coffee. I knew it would make me buzzy, and I'd end up a bit relapsed, but I needed the energy to do a few little chores, to take my mind off the hope-Ben-comes-home-safely-anxiety. And I wanted the house to look nice for his return.

11.53 a.m.    I hoped he had enjoyed coffee in a café in Bordeaux. And maybe a croissant. He likes coffee and a croissant. Especially a chocolate croissant.

11.54 a.m.    Fancied a chocolatey treat.

11.56 a.m.    Cut a tasty little slice of gateau for myself and gave Diamanda a big salmon treat, usually reserved for de-flea day – but today I felt she needed a special treat to cheer up her sad-cat eyes and missing-daddy ears. After salmon and gateau, we'd watch *Escape To The Chateau*.

11.57 a.m.   Did I feel some verse coming on?

11.58 a.m.   Yes!

*Salmon for my chat noir*
*I'm eating tasty gateau*
*Later we will both enjoy*
*Escape To The Chateau*

12.35 p.m.   Hurrah! A text.

HAD A WANDER ROUND VERY FRENCH SMELLING MARKET
AND BOUGHT GRUB FOR DINS THIS EVENING – NOW IN CAFE
HAVING LUNCH X

I smiled, knowing Ben was enjoying himself, and he
would have an excellent evening with fine wine and
delicious food, all nicely digested with good conversation. Then replied:

SOUNDS MAGNIFIQUE X

12.37 p.m.   Did I feel more verse coming on?........ I did.

*Ben has lunch in Bordeaux*
*He may visit the Place de la bourse*
*I fancy a chocolatey treat*
*Will I have more gateau?*

*Of course!*

1.05 p.m.   Diamanda and I enjoyed the peace while the workmen on the building site were at lunch. She curled
up next to me, approving of the Kitty Cat Tunic in
Joe Browns – red with a black cat design.

2.26 p.m.   I pecked away at a lovely late lunch of cottage cheese, Camembert, fresh crispy salad and French bread, like a hungry little vulture, as I perused Culture Vulture catalogue.

I enjoyed devouring photos of beautiful clothes, furniture and ornaments inspired by Russian folk art.... designs echoing traditional Kantha motifs from Bengali textiles.... oriental birds and flowers embracing the vibrancy of China and Japan.... and the bright designs inspired by New Mexico. But I much preferred the soft, cool colours of Scandinavia and the Scottish Highlands.

2.31 p.m.   The Christmas gift section at the end of the catalogue was the best bit. It made me look forward to the colours and sparkle of Christmas.... The Alpine Christmas decorations capturing the charm of a mountain Christmas from Innsbruck to Chamonix.... Italian gifts full of authentic flavours and scents to take you back to adventures from sunny Tuscany to the heart of Florence.... Eclectic gifts celebrating quintessentially British art and music.... But best of all I liked the French country gifts. Especially the tea towel celebrating the wealth of French bread and cheeses, the robe with a floral design recalling antique finds from Lyon, and Provence hand creams.

2.33 p.m.   While Diamanda admired the crème de la crème tote bag with a cat wearing a beret design, I wondered if Ben would bring me back a little French gift. Smelly French cheese would be nice.

4.02 p.m.   The workmen on the building site had ceased fire for the day, with their nail-guns and drilling. Phew! Peace at last. I could hear the birdies sing again, as

I leafed through Museum Selection catalogue, especially admiring the selection of ten robin paintings on Christmas cards, Winter Birds tea towel, Feeding Time candle (with blue tits, chaffinches, nuthatches and long-tailed tits in the winter snow design) and Robin Red Breast crackers.

There were some mini Christmas crackers with chocolate balls inside, and under the photo it said Christmas crackers are believed to have been invented by English confectioner Tom Smith. I'm sure Ben will be delighted to know this interesting piece of information.

He *was* delighted with the chocolate sprouts I gave him last Christmas from this catalogue, so will order them again – along with the selection of savoury biscuits for cheese (tomato and basil, mature cheddar, and Cheddar chilli), accompanied by a fruity trio of chutneys: sun-dried tomato and garlic, caramelised onion, and sweet chilli. Delicious.

4.12 p.m.  Perusing mouth-watering gifts is fun, but it's got to be....

4.13 p.m.  McVitie's time with a cuppa now, and a little perusal of the clothes in Museum Selection. The Impressionist socks – evoking paintings by Monet and Van Gogh, made me smile. So did the Art Nouveau cotton tunic and the Art Nouveau embroidered cape, William Morris jacket, and silk scarf based on botanical studies by painter Pierre Joseph Redoute. If I were a rich and famous artist I'd be floating around the house in theses creations, deep in arty thoughts.

The corduroy dress caught my eye. A delightful moss

green with pink embroidery on the button front. And I was interested to read that the term 'corduroy' was thought to derive from the French 'corde du roi', 'cord of the king'. I'm sure Ben will be enamoured by this wonderful piece of information.

5.00 p.m.     Diamanda and I planned our TV viewing for the evening. Tonight's episode of *Coronation Street* would be good. We'd find out what flattering business proposition Ray offers Michelle, if Emma lays her cards on the table for Steve, and if Bethany's setback sends Daniel on the warpath.

*Coronation Street* was to be followed by *Inside The Cockpit: The Concorde Crash*. On 25 July 2000, Concorde's perfect safety record went down in flames when mere minutes after take-off in Paris, Air France Flight 4590 crashed, killing 113 people. So what went wrong? Interviews with crash investigators, pilots, and air-traffic controllers working that day, tell the story.

5.03 p.m.     Diamanda sat on TV Weekly – don't look mummy!

5.04 p.m.     I decided to get an early night after *Grand Designs,* because Ben was catching his flight in the early hours. I wanted to be awake to receive his text message, telling me (hopefully) that all was well – he'd boarded his plane on time, then arrived safely at Gatwick airport. If I could get to sleep.

## Saturday 7th

4.27 a.m.     After finally falling asleep around one o'clock in the morning, I awoke after a horrible technicolour nightmare. I was at Gatwick airport waiting for Ben's plane to arrive. I stood on the runway and watched one plane after another appear out of the fog, coming in to land from the countries in my Culture Vulture catalogue. Russia.... India.... Scandinavia.... They were painted with the designs and colours of their country. They looked very beautiful and serene, until there was a BANG! BANG! BANG! – like the sound of the nail-guns on the building site. And the planes exploded. One after the other. There was a kaleido-scope of colour and matchstick bodies flying into the air with their heads on fire.

Vultures with rainbow plumage perched on the air-port roof. Vultures from many cultures – waiting, very still and silent, with sombre, salivating beaks, to pick at the bodies. I threw McVitie's chocolate biscuits and savoury biscuits onto the runway to distract them, but they didn't move. Just watched.

The plane from France appeared out of the fog, and there was another BANG! BANG! BANG! I tried to scream but no sound came out of my mouth. Then I awoke, heart pounding, and feeling panicky as I listened to the sad whistling sound of a plane flying over our town.

4.28 a.m.    My brain felt as foggy as Gatwick airport in my night-mare, my head felt hot, and I had a burning desire to send Ben a text message. But I didn't want to disturb him, he'd probably be at the airport, checking in now.

4.30 a.m.    I wondered why the Concorde crashed so soon after taking off from Paris in 2000.

4.31 a.m.    The weather felt even colder today.

4.32 a.m.    The world was a cold, dark, scary place.

4.34 a.m.    Time to snuggle up in my big fluffy dressing gown, with a nice warm milky drink, nice chocolate biscuit, nice warm cat, and Jane McDonald who is always nice, in a repeat of *Cruising With Jane McDonald*.

4.54 a.m.    Watching the cruiser cruising along is..... so.... very relaxing.

Feel so sleepy... will lie down for a moment on sofa.

My eyes are closing...

I'm dozing off..

To sea.

4.59 a.m.    I'm on the cruiser with Jane, enjoying afternoon tea with chocolate biscuits...

5.00 a.m.    But a storm is brewing and soon becomes raging....

5.01 a.m.    Massive waves...

5.02 a.m.    I fall overboard...

5.03 a.m.    Down...

5.04 a.m.    Down...

5.05 a.m.    Into the icy cold sea...

5.06 a.m.    My ears are ringing.
I wake up.

Is this really happening?

Ooh, got a text!

SAFELY THROUGH CUSTOMS AND CHECK IN AT AIRPORT
AND PLANE ON TIME AT THE MOMENT X

I replied:

OH GOOD - HOPE THERE'S NO DELAY X

5.15 a.m.   Time for nice cuppa and nice choccy biscuit with
Ann Maurice, who is always nice, in a repeat of
*House Doctor*.

5.40 a.m.   I listen to a plane flying overhead and wonder if
Ben has boarded his plane yet.

5.42 a.m.   Another text!

SITTING IN IꓱC AWAITING TAKE OFF

I reply:

BON VOYAGE X

\* \* \* \* \* \* \* \*

5.46 p.m.   Sitting on the bed, staring at the sky (what little bit
of sky I can see now, above the flats). It's starting to
get light. I watch a plane fly overhead. Planes look
so very tiny when they are high in the sky, but so
very big when you climb on board one.

I don't like the thought of Ben, high in the sky. Do I
feel some verse coming on about planes that fly so
high in the sky, and the thought of Ben up there,
making me want to cry?...... No, not today.

5.47 p.m.    Diamanda's snoring makes me want to laugh, but I mustn't wake her up. I say a little get-home-safely-Ben-and-family prayer in my head.

\* \* \* \* \* \* \* \*

7.18 a.m.    Had a horrible thought. Ben should land soon, but what if, come nine o'clock, I haven't heard from him? Should I text him? Yes. If he doesn't answer should I ring the airport? Yes.

7.19 a.m.    Feel...

7.20 a.m.    So...

7.22 a.m.    Tired...

7.24 a.m.    Eyes drooping...

7.26 a.m.    I'm falling...

7.27 a.m.    Falling...

7.28 a.m.    Out of a plane...

7.29 a.m.    Through fluffy white clouds...

7.30 a.m.    The sky is full of ringing bells. Am I with the angels?

I wake up. That's my phone. Where's my phone?

Where is it?

Can't find it *anywhere.*

7.31 a.m.    WHERE IS MY PHONE!?

## WHERE... IS... MY... PHONE!!!!????

My plodding around, moving things and muttering to myself, wakes up Diamanda. She yawns, stretches, and pads off for a snack and a drink. I pick up my phone, beautifully warmed from a cat body sleeping on it, and read the message.

JUST LANDED AT GATWICK X

\* \* \* \* \* \* \* \*

9.22 a.m.

BEN:      Close your eyes.

ME:       OK.

BEN:      Both eyes?

ME:       Yes (closing right eye).

BEN:      Hold out your paws.

ME:       Feels light.

BEN:      Open eyes.

ME:       Oh, what gorgeous autumnal colours. *Seupair!*

BEN:      I thought you'd like it.

ME:       Love the crimson grapes and orangy-mustard vine leaf design around the illustrations of places to visit in Bordeaux....Le grande théâtre.... Porte Cailhou.... La Ponte de Pierre.... Palace de la bourse – did you go there?

BEN:     Oui! I'll show you the photos later.

ME:      BON!....... I like all the little barrels among the vine
         leaves with the names of wines from Bordeaux. Côtes
         de Castillon... Pressac Léognan... Saint Épstèphe...
         Moulis... Medoc, there's so many..... over twenty! I
         thought all wine from Bordeaux was called Bordeaux!

BEN:     It will look good on our newly painted kitchen wall.
         Go with the French café and street scenes.

ME:      OUI!.... It's funny, I was admiring a tea towel with a
         French design yesterday, with a French bread and
         cheese design. But this is a much better one. *Merci
         beaucoup monsiuer!*

BEN:     Close your eyes again.

ME:      Ooh (giggling).

BEN:     No need to put your paws out, just sniff.

ME:      **MON DIEU!**... Odeur forte!

BEN:     Open eyes.

ME:      I can't see what it is in the wrapper but I guess, from
         the HUGE PONG and the weight, it's a beautiful big
         lump of French cheese! I know it'll be delicious.

BEN:     Oui madame.

ME:      So glad you are home, safe and sound.

Is this really happening?

BEN:      Moi aussi!

* * * * * * * *

*Smell is the sense of memory and desire.*

Jean-Jacques Rousseau

**eight months and twenty-three days later**

# June

## Monday 1st

BEN: My hay fever is driving me nuts! I know we've got a slot with Tesco tomorrow evening, but I can't wait till then for my Loratadine tablets. Must have them today!

ME: I can understand that, you do look like you are sufferin'........ Loratadine reminds me – I must find my labradorite.

BEN: Is that a remedy for Labrador breath?

ME: It's a crystal! I need it for another spell I'm doing to help protect family, friends and us from the carnivorous monster.

BEN: I take you mean the coronavirus monster, because you don't like the word (laughing).

ME: You know me too well. I prefer the word coronation because –

BEN: You're a fan of *Coronation Street?*

ME: Correct! And Cornetto.

BEN: Your fave ice cream.

ME: Cornflower.

BEN: Fave flower.

ME: Cornucopia.

BEN: Erm....

ME: An abundance of good things – like when we get a delivery from a supermarket....... Anyway, I've got angelite, smokey quartz, and turquoise howite crystals, candles for protection and a seashell for my spell work.

BEN: Great. I'm off into town now. Is there anything I can get you to help with your spell work? Angel cakes? Special herbs? Silvery string? Turquoise ribbon?

ME: Chocolatey fairy cakes would be good.

BEN: Essential for witchery?

ME: *Most certainly!* Helps with mental and physical energy. The only thing is, I need a few strands of hair from all our friends and family.

BEN: I can just imagine you writing to everyone requesting a few strands off hair (laughing).

ME: They wouldn't be surprised!.... But I think I'll use a photo instead or carve their name on a candle.

BEN: Sealed with snail slime?

ME: I'm sure a snail would be happy to oblige. They know all about protecting themselves in a lovely shell.

BEN: So it's just fairy cakes then.

ME: Oh, we need freezer bags, so I can freeze some veg, in case we can't get the veg we ordered.

BEN:    OK.

ME:    And if Tesco substitutes a small loaf of wholemeal with a large one, I'll freeze some slices.

BEN:    Good idea.

ME:    Hope people will be social distancing in the shops. A woman went into a supermarket –

BEN:    Is this a joke?

ME:    No dear. I was listening to her on a phone-in on Radio Kent. She said she was in a supermarket a few days ago and no-one was distancing. *Is this really happening?*

BEN:    Yeah.

ME:    I must stop listening to phone-ins. There's so many sad stories, it's getting me down. But it is *very heart warming* when after a caller tells the radio presenter of their predicament, lots of people email or phone the station to offer their services. I always shed a tear or three.

BEN:    What are you like (sneezing and sniffing).

ME:    I could make you a lovely infusion of nettle juice for you to sip, to help with your symptoms. And slice some cold cucumber to lay on your eyes.

BEN:    No thanks. No witchy remedies for me! And I prefer cucumber in a sandwich. Must have my tablets. I'll be careful in Sainsbury's and wear my gloves.

ME: I think masks will become compulsory if things get worse. My witchy senses feel it will happen. Oh, and I heard a woman say on the radio that wearing a face mask helped her hay fever.

BEN: I've bought masks for us with a colourful cat design.

ME: Oh, good! The black ones will make us look like we're about to rob a bank, and the blue or white ones will make us feel like we are about to cut into a body to perform an operation. I haven't left the house since Christmas, but I may need one in future. I saw on *The Ellen DeGeneres Show* what some people are wearing in American supermarkets – *so funny!*

BEN: Do enlighten me.

ME: Halloween costumes, covering their body and face. Which I think is great – lightens the mood of these horrible times. Also suits of armour, diving gear with a snorkel, and the one I liked best was a pink unicorn. How can you not laugh when you are shopping with a pink unicorn!.... You could wear the pirate's costume I made you for Pirate's Day in Hastings years ago – the white blouse with black lace-up front, black shorts with ragged legs, and the black banana, I mean bandanna, with white skull and crossbones design, over your nose! I know where they are, second drawer in the chest of drawers under the bedroom window. I got you a toy parrot to sit on your shoulder too and a plastic cutlass. Remember?

BEN: Yes dear.

ME: The plastic cutlass looks very realistic, so you could

threaten people if they come too close, especially if they are coughing and sneezing! And you do a really good *AH, HARRRRRRR!!!!!!* pirate impression. I vividly recall the time you sat, bolt upright in your sleep, made the pirate noise, said 'Pieces of eight' loudly, then fell back down to sleep. You didn't remember in the morning. Scared the bloomin' life out of me (giggling).

BEN:    Thank you for reminding me about that dear. No time to dress up as a pirate now – must go!

ME:    Non essential shops are open today.

BEN:    Yeah.

ME:    I'm wondering if people will be flocking into town after the lockdown.

BEN:    Like bats out of hell!

ME:    Or prisoners escaping from prison. Carol on *Loose Women* calls lockdown, lock-up. It was nice meeting her many moons ago before she was famous, she had a lovely friendly aura.

BEN:    Yeah, she did!

ME:    I expect a lot of young people will be out and about and the very old folk will stay at home. I feel for them. But it's good to know there are so many people willing to help them.

BEN:    Yeah, it is.

ME:    I can't help feeling the lifting of the lockdown is too soon, even if it's good for the economy. Hopefully people will social distance and wash their hands, but you only had to see the gatherings of young families during lockdown on the low income estate next to our street, to know that a lot of people –

BEN: Won't give a monkeys!

ME: Yes. But on a good note, I'm *so glad* we're able to order everything we need online. And I'm grateful for the food we've been able to get, even if some things are substituted.

BEN: Me too.

ME: Actually, we've had some good substitutes from ASDA haven't we. Things we never thought to try, but will buy again!

BEN: True, when we can get a slot.

ME: I know. And I think *more and more* people will be going online, so it'll not get easier. But I'm going to do what Wendy of Weekly Wife suggested for a happier life.

BEN: I can't wait to hear.

ME: Make a gratitude list. She says writing a gratitude list focuses your mind on the positive aspects of your life, making you feel better. You should write one too.

BEN: Must I? Can't you write it for me?

ME: OK..... First on *your* list will be, you are fortunate to have a partner who likes to focus on the positive aspects of her life.

BEN: Lucky me! Right I'm off.

ME: First on *my* list – I'm fortunate to have a partner who does the shopping.

BEN: Anything else you'd like from Sainsbury's?

ME: I'll have to think for a moment. There are a few things we've not been able to get online when we last had a slot, and Tesco may not have them in stock. Erm...

BEN: Text me. You'll remember as soon as I'm out the door.

ME: Did you know Sainsbury's is Britain's oldest supermarket?

BEN: That's interesting. You can add to my gratitude list – I have a *most informative* partner.

ME: Will do!

\* \* \* \* \* \* \* \*

11.23 a.m. I send Ben a text message:

CAN YOU GET THE SOUPS I LIKE AND THE WATER BISCUITS YOU LIKE PLZ

Ben replied:

WILL DO – SAW A SIGN ON CASH MACHINE SAYING ALL NOTES IN MACHINE HAD BEEN QUARANTINED FOR 72

HOURS – 50 DEFINITELY VIRUS FREE

11.25 a.m.    I replied:

THAT'S GOOD – HOPE THEY WERE WELL LOOKED AFTER IN THE MONEY HOTEL

Ben replied:

WHAT ARE YOU LIKE

\* \* \* \* \* \* \* \*

12.46 p.m.

ME:        You were *ages* in town. I was getting a little worried.

BEN:       There was a long queue at the cash machine and Sainsbury's.

ME:        Were people social distancing?

BEN:       Yeah. And they were very good in Sainsbury's with the precautions.

ME:        That's a relief. If you get the virus it'll be horrid for you. And with my M.E. and asthma, I'll probably be a goner if I contract it from you.

BEN:       It's a relief to have my hay fever relief.

ME:        I'm relieved you are relieved that you have your hay fever relief.

WE LAUGH

## Tuesday 2nd

BEN:    Why are you washing your dressing gown in the bath?

ME:     I'm not washing it. I've just been soaking it in warm water and rubbing away the odd stain – don't want to put it on a hot wash in the washing machine. I memorised where the little stains were, because when clothes are in water you can't see marks so clearly. I knew where the soup stains were – close to a pink flower on the neckline, and about knee length on the front, next to a purple flower. The coffee stain was on the left pocket on a yellow flower. And –

BEN:    There's more?

ME:     Oh yes. There were two tiny dark specks, one on the left sleeve near the green leaf of a purple flower, and one on the belt, on a green leaf of a pink flower. I hoped they weren't black acrylic paint specks that hadn't come out in previous washes. But they came out easily so I guessed they were tiny flakes of plain chocolate.

BEN:    What fun you have.

ME:     It *was fun* when I gently swirled the dressing gown round and round in the bath. It sort of rippled like a beautiful pink, purple, yellow, leaf green and sky blue sea creature, the belt – like the tentacles of an octopus. I imagined I was swimming with it, deep in the ocean.

BEN:    Did you sing a Beatles song, about wanting to be

under the sea in an octopus's garden?

ME:      I did!

         *I'd like to be under the sea*
         *In an octopus's garden in the shade*
         *He'd let us in, knows where we've been*
         *In his octopus's garden in the shade*

         Can you play it on your guitar so I can sing along?

BEN:     Yep.

ME:      I'll let the bath water out now. Would you mind wringing my dressing gown out for me and putting it in the washing machine, it's *SO HEAVY* when it's wet.

BEN:     OK.

ME:      You can imagine you're wringing our P. M.'s neck.

BEN:     It will be a pleasure.

                    * * * * * * * *

ME:      There's a programme on tonight about the Heinz baked bean factory in Wigan. With COVID 19 triggering a rush on tinned goods, the factory has nearly doubled production to almost fifty million cans a month. *Fifty million!* Human beings are going to be full of beans. They will become human –

BEN:     Beans!

ME:      I'm looking forward to *Coronation Street* tomorrow night because Shona is going to spill the beans.

BEN:     All this talk of beans is making me want egg, chips, and beans from our stash of Heinz beans tonight.

ME:      Sounds good. We seem to be eating more since the lockdown. I texted my sister a few days ago and she said her family have been eating more too.

BEN:     I'm putting on weight (looking a little grim).

ME:      Me too. We'll blame it on the lockdown..... I've got a Michael Jackson song to cheer you up.

         *Don't blame it on the sunshine*
         *Don't blame it on the moonlight*
         *Don't blame it on the good time*
         *Blame it on the lockdown*

BEN:     *I just can't, I just can't*
         *I just can't control my appetite*

                    WE LAUGH

BEN:     Heinz beans on toast for lunch?

ME:      Yes! I'd love to be full of beans. I'll stick some bread in the toaster.

BEN:     I'll crack open a can.

ME:      A presenter on Radio Kent said his clothes were getting very tight now (placing two slices of bread in toaster). People will have exercised less during the lockdown, and with the stress and comfort eating, many like us will have gained pounds. Though fortunately we're not too stressed.

BEN:     People will need to get to the shops for bigger sized clothes, or order online.

ME:      Or go on a diet. There will probably be a big demand for slimming products like Slimfast. I think I'll just cut down on the bread after today (taking bread out of toaster and placing two more slices in). What will you cut down on?

BEN:     Dunno. Nothing yet. Will have mushrooms, tomatoes and sausages with my egg, chips and beans tonight (laughing).

ME:      Maybe when you go for your walk tomorrow, it should be a jog around the park. Twice!

BEN:     Yes dear.

\* \* \* \* \* \* \* \*

ME:      The sound of the ice cream van playing the tune from the old Cornetto advert, is making me fancy just one –

BEN:     Cornetto (bursting into song).

         *Just one Cornetto*
         *Give it to me!*

ME:      *There's a pandemic*
         *We need a treat!*

\* \* \* \* \* \* \* \*

ME:      A sound of screeching breaks just now, didn't sound good. I was waiting for the awful sound of a crash.

BEN:       Me too.

ME:        I'm glad there wasn't a crash. Accidents involving an ice cream van are very tragic.

BEN:       Why's that?

ME:        Because hundreds and thousands are lost.

BEN:       What are you like.

\* \* \* \* \* \* \* \* \*

1.20 p.m.

BEN:       You look chilled out.

ME:        I've been sitting in the garden with my Cornetto, wiggling my toes to use up some calories, and enjoying the sound of the wind in the trees and the buzzy buzzing bees, and I've just de-flead Diamanda, so she has no fleas.

BEN:       I can hear some verse coming on.

ME:        *The wind in the trees*
           *And the buzzy buzzing bees*
           *I've just de-flead our pussy*

BEN:       *And he thinks he's going to sneeze*

ME:        I shall entitle our verse, *Man with hay fever who enjoys his food and lots of it!*

\* \* \* \* \* \* \* \* \*

ME:    I've just read in Weekly Wife, six storks hatched in
       West Sussex this Spring. They were the first born in
       Britain for six hundred years. Isn't that sweet.

BEN:   Very nice dear.

ME:    I remember when my little brother was born, when
       I was five, and we were sent a card with a stork
       carrying a baby. And I recall a small cake with baby
       blue and white icing, and a beautiful tiny stork on
       top, carrying a baby in its beak. I was entranced with
       the idea, and gently rocked the baby when mum
       wasn't looking.

BEN:   I imagine a lot of young mums wish their baby was
       delivered by a stork.

ME:    Lots of storks may be needed at the end of this year.

BEN:   Why?

ME:    There could be a baby boom after the lockdown,
       like there was after World War Two started, and the
       power cuts in the seventies. Remember the power
       cuts?

BEN:   Yeah.

* * * * * * * *

ME:    Do you remember Stork margarine?

BEN:   I do!

ME:    I wonder why it was called Stork. Do you know why
       Bird's custard powder is called Bird's?

BEN:         Nope, but I'm sure you're going to tell me.

ME:          It was invented by Alfred Bird in eighteen thirty-seven, to cater for his wife's egg allergy.

BEN:         That was nice of him.

* * * * * * * *

ME:          The animation *Storks* is on tonight. I think I'll watch it while you are working on your music. Shall we have *baby* carrots and *baby* spinach leaves with dinner tonight?

BEN:         Don't get *carried* away!... I don't think carrots and spinach will go with egg, chips and beans.

ME:          Oh! I forgot what we'd decided to have for dinner. We could have button mushrooms and tiny cherry tomatoes.

BEN:         Anything you say dear.

* * * * * * * *

ME:          The first birth on a plane occurred in nineteen twenty-nine and was planned by the father. The plane circled at two thousand feet until baby Airleen arrived. What a strange thing to do! What did she put as place of birth on her passport?... *I've no idea, I was very high at the time?*.... Or, *I can't answer that question, I'm above all that?*

BEN:         She probably lived her life with her head in the clouds, enjoying the high life.

ME:        Was always on another plane.

BEN:       And enjoying little flights of fancy.

ME:        Always the height of fashion.

BEN:       Never felt grounded....... You've got that look, I can see a story coming on!

ME:        She became an air hostess and fell in love with a handsome pilot. They married, and one day he brought her down to earth during a terrible storm, when the plane was struck by lightening. They were lucky to survive. She was pregnant at the time, and the stress almost made her go into early labour. When she gave birth to a baby girl, they named her Storm – like Ronan Keating's wife. Then one day, years later, she found out her wealthy father had paid her husband a small fortune to take her on a flight during a storm, in the hope that his first grand-child would be born on a plane. So she divorced her husband, never spoke to her father again, and re-named her child Verity, because Verity means truth.

WE LAUGH

7.22 p.m.   Ben is playing his guitar.

ME:        That's lovely. What you are playing?

BEN:       *Summer Breeze* by the Isley Brothers.

ME:        *Summer breeze makes me feel fine*
           *Blowing through the jasmine in my mind*

           Beautiful song.

\* \* \* \* \* \* \* \*

ME:    It makes me sad, that just when you got your act together with a *really good* set of songs and melodies, and started to get gigs, the pandemic happened (deep sigh). And the lovely restaurant owner, Franco, who was giving you gigs, had only just started up his business, and was doing well. I *so feel* for everyone in hospitality. And musicians. *Everyone* working in the entertainment industry (very deep sigh). And I feel the carnivorous monster is going to be with us for quite a while. A long while.

BEN:    Is this really happening?

ME:    I'm afraid so. And sometimes I'm so afraid. Not just for me – for our family and friends, especially those most vulnerable. I get days when I want to contact all my family and friends to ask if they are OK. Well, every few days really. At the moment, thankfully they are all fine. I contacted them all a couple of days ago.

We must try to think of the positives. How much people are helping those in need. Listen to music and sing songs we love, find new hobbies, learn to love jigsaw puzzles – to keep our spirits up.

BEN:    I'll leave that to you dear.

ME:    Wendy of Weekly Wife says that now more than ever we need a creative outlet, whether it's painting, knitting or yoga. Did you know something repetitive or rhythmic will help your mind unwind and release stress? We should think of this as giving our head a hug. Would you like a head hug?

BEN:        Yeah!

*  *  *  *  *  *  *  *

8.17 p.m.

BEN:        We've got a Tesco delivery arriving soon.

ME:         I've had my M.E. eyeballs in. When you printed out the shopping list for me to see if I wanted to add anything, I read Farmhouse Wholemeal Loaf, as *Famous* Wholemeal Loaf. Fair Trade bananas as *Fairytale* bananas. Reduced fat hummus as reduced fat *humans*. Then, Meat Free Pasties as Meat Free *Parasites*. Where it said, Updated Order Confirmation, I read this as *Update and Order Your Coffin!*... I'm wondering if the pandemic is getting to me a little. Reading an advert for an insurance company that said they guarantee to pay every claim, I read this as, *We quarantine to pay every claim*. And in TV Weekly I read the film *Look Who's Talking* as *Lockdown Talking*.

BEN:        There probably will be a film in the future with that title.

8.33 p.m.

BEN:        Sounds like the Tesco van!

ME:         That will be the Famous Wholemeal Loaf, Fairytale Bananas and Meat Free Parasites.

BEN:        And a coffin!

ME:         I'll give you a hand.

BEN:     Mustn't tire yourself.

8.36 p.m.

ME:      I'll just put away the light stuff (picking up the toilet rolls, kitchen rolls and toothpaste). I must put having enough loo rolls on my gratitude list.

BEN:     They didn't have bananas. I'll get some tomorrow.

ME:      *Yes, we have no bananas*
         *We have-a no bananas today*

BEN:     Oh, she's off!

ME:      *We've string beans and onions*
         *Cabbages and scallions*
         *And all sorts of fruit and say*
         *We have an old fashioned to-ma-to*
         *A long Island po-tah-to*
         *But yes, we have no bananas*
         *We have no bananas today!*

## Wednesday 3rd

11.50 p.m.   Ben returns from visiting his friends Rob and Sally.

BEN:     Here you are, lots of lovely home-grown fresh veg.

ME:      Oh, *how generous!*

BEN:     Runner beans, beetroot and onions.

ME:      Cucumber *and* tomatoes.

*We've got runner beans and onions*
*Cucumber and tomatoes*
*And beetroot for a lovely salad day*
*And yes we'll have more bananas*
*We'll have more bananas today!*

I'm going to add veg from friends to my gratitude list.

BEN:    You do that dear.

ME:     I'm grateful too, *very grateful* that dad's not in a care home, the way things are. And he has his lovely lady carers, Bella and Laura, to do his shopping and health care.

BEN:    And a kind neighbour, Lynn, pops in to do house-work for him. He rang and left a message, I'll call him back later.

ME:     I must write and thank Lynn..... My brother is doing OK, though London is not the best place to live at the moment. Probably one of the worst. He said it's hard to social distance on public transport.

BEN:    I can imagine.

ME:     I feel fortunate I'm not a nurse or doctor working in a hospital. They must be exhausted, and concerned about catching the virus themselves. I had a night-mare about doctors and nurses getting ill one by one, they were collapsing in the hospital corridors. And at the same time, patients who were ill with the virus were being brought in, and had to be treated in the corridors because the wards were full. The whole dream was the same blue and white as surgical

302

masks, then it all started turning blood red and –

BEN: You should have a break from watching the news dear. By the way, your big rainbow drawing with a thank you to the NHS looks good in the window. I like the way it arches across three little window panes.

ME: Thanks! Took a bit of working out to get the arch just right. I consulted one of the rainbow photos I took from our bedroom window. The sun is fading the colours now, so I'll have to brighten them up. My felt-tips are drying up, can you order or get me a new pack?

BEN: Will do.

ME: Great. I love a nice pack of new felt-tip pens, and a nice colouring-in session. Especially in my Harry Potter colouring-in book......... I think the rainbow drawings by children are the best, don't you – so charming. Like the one in the window at the end of George Street, done by a wee girl. I noticed it when I went outside to admire my own creation!

BEN: Yeah, I saw it. It *is* charming.

ME: I must make another sign to put on the front door to thank our lovely postman, the bin men, and delivery people.

BEN: What happened to the other one?

ME: The strong winds and rain blew it off the nail on the front door. I thought I'd waterproofed it *really well* with cling film and sellotape, but once it was on the path outside next door, the rain seeped in and it was looking rather sad – all runny black letters, like a teenage girl wearing lots of mascara, who has wept all day after splitting-up with her boyfriend. They had been together *two whole weeks* and she'd already planned their wedding, chosen the names of the five children they would have, and where they'd live.

The rainbow edges were like the sad teenage girl's orangy-red lipstick and greeny-blue eyeshadow, smeared all over her cheeks as she sobs and wipes it all away. I'm tempted to keep the edges because they look quite arty – and do fresh lettering!

BEN:        Good idea dear.

1.47 p.m.

ME:        I've just watched the lunchtime news. I'm *SO GLAD* we're not stuck on a cruise ship, where people are getting ill and having to self-isolate. I feel ill just thinking about it. I was quite annoyed when I heard a caller on Radio Kent saying she had a cruise booked, was thinking of cancelling, and the cruise people offered her one hundred pounds spending money if she didn't cancel....... *Here's one hundred pounds – please come aboard, risk your life, end up self-isolating in fear in your cabin, and enjoy the holiday of your nightmares, paid for with your life savings, after working hard all your life, so we don't lose your custom.*

BEN:        You need to have a break from listening to Radio Kent.

ME:        I know, *I know*....... Lets talk about dinner. Veggie

304

burgers with lots of *beautifully delicious* home grown veg?

BEN:      Sounds good to me!

1.50 p.m.

ME:      That tune you're playing sounds nice. What is it?

BEN:      *The Way You Look Tonight,* by Jerome Kern and Dorothy Fields. It was first sung by Fred Astaire to Ginger Rogers in the film, *The Swing,* back in nineteen thirty-six. He sang it from another room while she was in the bathroom washing her hair.

ME:      That's a lovely old song. The baby Airleen would have been seven years old in nineteen thirty-six.

BEN:      Airleen?

ME:      The story I made up yesterday, after reading about a baby born on a plane, which was planned by her father in –

BEN:      Nineteen twenty-nine!..... You've got that look again. Do I feel another story coming on? Or a song? Or a poem?

ME:      All three if you're lucky.

BEN:      Shall I put the kettle on for coffee and story time?

ME:      Good idea.

1.56 p.m.

ME:          Are you sitting comfortably?

BEN:        Yep.

ME:          Airleen's father would sing *The Way You Look Tonight* to her mother when they were getting ready to go out for dinner. That was in happier days before she divorced him, because he not only insisted she give birth to Airleen during a flight, but also Airleen's four siblings – three girls; Louisiana, Maryland and Georgia, and one boy – Kentucky.

BEN:        Who ate too much fried chicken!

ME:          Yes! And you can guess which country they were flying over.

BEN:        With all those kids to care for there must've been a lot of *Washington*.

WE LAUGH

2.21 p.m.

ME:          I was in the garden just now and overheard the neighbours talking. Our new young neighbours at number six were taking to their young neighbours at number five. The women were saying how much they'd been looking forward to the shops opening.

BEN:        You ladies must have your retail therapy.

ME:          Like Diamanda enjoys her rub-tail therapy.

BEN: Yeah.

ME: We're so lucky to have friendly and pleasant new neighbours on both sides now. And the view of the flats opposite, now they are built, isn't as bad as I thought it would be. Not so close, because of the car parking spaces, that I watched being beautifully paved with pale grey bricks, one by one, by hand. I can still see the workmen in my mind's eye, working painstakingly, and I wanted to call out of the window 'Lovely job you guys!' Because I could see how tired and back achy they were feeling.

BEN: You should have.

ME: It looks like an architect's drawing brought to life with the shrubs – different shades of green, between the parking spaces, and four saplings – one opposite our house, one on a nice patch of very green grass on the corner, and two further down the street. It makes me smile after all those years I spent in a drawing office.

BEN: Did you draw housing developments?

ME: Sort of. I would get drawings of housing developments from architects, reduce them in size, then draw them onto maps, so I could plot the gas mains mains. I never saw the completed estates, just the the foundations when I measured-up where the gas mains were – nice bit of 63mm low pressure PE pipe here, bit of 250mm medium pressure PE pipe going in there.

BEN: Was it a *high pressure* job?

ME: Sometimes (giggling) when a job was urgent!

BEN: It makes me laugh, the times we've been out, when you've felt the urge to get out of the car and measure-up when you see British Gas roadworks. And you tell me the size of the pipes you see at the side of the road, and how far you estimate they will be from the kerb.

ME: Yes, it gave us a bit of a laugh!......... I thought during the lockdown the shrubs, trees, and bits of lawn would be neglected, but they've been very well looked after. So, though I've lost my view, the front parking bit of the flats looks better than the plain, grey car park with lots of boring cars and dull, falling apart fencing.

BEN: Yeah.

\* \* \* \* \* \* \* \*

6.10 p.m. Ben is in the bath. I sing to him from the bedroom.

ME: *Some day, when I'm awfully low*
*When the world is cold*
*I will feel a glow just thinking of you*
*And the way you look tonight*

6.14 p.m. Ben walks into the bedroom rubbing his hair with a towel. I make up a little song, to the same tune.

ME: *I think, it's time I cut your hair*
*Snip without a care*
*Trimming with the flare of a hairdresser*
*So you don't look a fright tonight*

BEN: Yeah (glancing in the mirror), it's time you gave me

another haircut.

ME: I can't believe how fast your hair grows! I'm happy to give you another trim, but the hairdressers open on the fifteenth, wouldn't you rather wait till then?

BEN: No, you're doing a good job.

ME: Well, I do my best! It's nice you don't mind me and my little paws getting tired and only cutting one side one day, then another side another day.

BEN: The back another day. You can put cutting my hair on my gratitude list.

ME: It's my biggest challenge since painting the spooky Mona Lisa cat. I've never cut anyone's hair before! I've always been in awe of hairdressers. I spent most of my working life at a drawing board and could erase my mistakes, but if you cut someone's hair wrong, you can't stick it back on. Or if you frazzle it, it's hard to un-frazzle. Heat can kill hair!... I was dead nervous about cutting your hair, but now I'm amazed at how much I enjoy it – your head feels like my little sculpture that I want to perfect. And I love the sound of the sharp scissors snipping away. Brings to mind the lovely sort of grinding sound of sharp scissors cutting thick, good quality material when you're making curtains. You know the sound?

BEN: Can't say I do.

ME: Men who haven't got a partner to cut their hair, and don't feel able to cut it themselves, are going to have lockdown hair. Long and floppy like in the seventies. It will match the seventies fashions that are back. You had long, bushy hair back then didn't you.

BEN: Yeah.

ME: You now have C.B.P. hair.

BEN: C.B.P?

ME: Cut by partner hair.

WE LAUGH

## Thursday 4th

9.22 a.m.

ME: I'd love a day out. An afternoon at the seaside.

BEN: I'm not surprised. You haven't left the house since visiting your family at Christmas.

ME: I could do with some sea air. Do us both good. From what I've seen on the news, people are not social distancing on beaches, but I think that may be at popular places like Hastings and Whitstable. We should go to a sleepy seaside town, like the one we went to when we viewed the Oyster House.

BEN: Yeah, Pevensey Bay.

ME: And now the shops are open and people are back at work, there will be fewer people on the beach in the week. Hopefully.

BEN: We could go to Pevensey tomorrow if you're up to it. The weather forecast looks good.

ME: I am! In my stars, Cosmic Colin said time spent resting and relaxing will recharge your batteries and leave you raring to go. He is right. I have been resting a lot, and my batteries are charged, as much as they can be. Mostly mentally! But I can't wait! *CAN'T WAIT* to be beside the seaside!

*Oh, I can't wait to be beside the seaside*
*Oh, I can't wait to be beside the sea*
*I can't wait to be beside the prom, prom, prom*
*When the band all play tiddely om pom, pom*

BEN: I'll have to see if the car is still going.

ME: Oh, yes. You've not driven anywhere since the lockdown.

\* \* \* \* \* \* \* \*

9.44 a.m.

ME: Is the car OK?

BEN: The engine started running first time.

ME: Wonderful!

10.24 a.m.

BEN: That's a nice little smile on your face.

ME: I was thinking of something else to add to my gratitude list. I feel happy that *Coronation Street* is filmed weeks and weeks ahead – so the programme didn't just stop when we had lockdown. And they are continuing to film, which is great.

BEN: I'm happy for you dear.

ME: And I'm happy for us that Diamanda makes us smile every day. You know when *Coronation Street* starts and there's the sound of a cat meow as a ginger cat climbs down from a roof?

BEN: I haven't noticed the cat. Or the meow.

ME: Well, the cat *is* only fleeting as it jumps down from a roof, and it's a quiet meow, behind the loud trumpety music. Anyway, last night Diamanda was sitting with me watching the programme, and when the cat meowed, she meowed back. Isn't that sweet.

BEN: Don't tell me, she's a fan too.

ME: Of course. And I'm a fan of Bill Roache now.

BEN: Bill who?

ME: He plays Ken Barlow.

BEN: Oh, yeah.

ME: He was in the very first episode sixty years ago – well it'll be sixty years in December.

BEN: He must be getting on a bit now.

ME: He's eighty-eight, and still in *Corrie!* And he's in Guinness World Records for being the longest-serving TV soap star.

BEN: Marvellous. I expect you're a fan of Roy too, who runs the cafe, Roy's Rolls, because he's always full of interesting facts.

ME: I am (smiling).

1.05 p.m.

ME: I'm going to miss clapping for carers tonight – showing appreciation for our brave, hard working NHS.

BEN: Yeah.

ME: My paws can't clap – I'm a bit clapped-out these days! But it was fun using my percussion instruments instead. And it was nice, you clapping at the front door, and me leaning out of the bedroom window, trying not to drop my percussion instruments onto the pavement, or an unsuspecting passer by!

BEN: The claves and cow bells sounded good.

ME: I liked seeing the neighbours at their front doors and this feeling of we're all in this together. One time you were at the front door, and instead of making a din with my percussion, I went out into the garden. As we're a bit high up I could hear the noise rising up from the houses in our town, getting louder and louder – lots of clanking of saucepans as well as clapping and cheering. Made me so –

BEN: You came indoors with a soggy sheet of kitchen roll screwed up in your hand.

ME: Two sheets! It was more emotional than when we went to see the London Symphony Orchestra, and I silently wept through most of the performance. The clap for carers was the people of Maidstone's symphony of gratitude – starting off with a few claps and taps, then reaching a wonderful crescendo for ten minutes.

BEN: I quite agree dear.

\* \* \* \* \* \* \* \*

1.43 p.m.

BEN: Dare I ask why you are wearing a pair of your knickers over your face?

ME: It makes a pretty, lacy face mask, with the leg holes for my eyes. And the material is thinner. The face mask you got is a sweet, cat pattern, but the layers of cotton are *so thick,* I feel I can't breathe.

BEN: I'll get you a thinner one.

ME: OK, thanks. But it would be fun to go into a shop with my knickers on my head – It's the only time people will think it acceptable, and it would give them a laugh. Maybe someone from a local news-paper would see me and take a photo, and put me on the front page, *and then* I'll be on the local news and start a trend!

2.06 p.m.

BEN: I'm going to put petrol in the car. Want anything in town?

ME:       I'll give you a little list, I thought I'd sort a nice picnic for tomorrow.

BEN:     Great!

ME:       *Oh, I do like to be beside the seaside*
*Oh, I do like to be beside the sea*
*Oh, I do like to be beside the prom, prom, prom*

BEN:     *When the band all play tiddely om pom, pom*

## Thursday 5th

12.45 p.m.

BEN:     Ready to go?

ME:       Yes! Got my seaside hoodie in case it gets chilly. Sunglasses, cotton gloves for protection when in the public toilets, cotton knickers to wear on head.

BEN:     You're not going to wear your knickers on your head are you?

ME:       Only joking. Got a cool box packed with lovely picnic grub, and a cat full of tuna treat – to keep her happy while we're out. Me, full of glee for a day by the sea. There may be queues at the toilets so I'd better have a wee.

BEN:     Feel a poem coming on?

ME:       Not yet. Maybe later.

BEN:     Car full of petrol. Festival chairs in boot.

ME: Wearing knickers on my head would give everyone a hoot.

12.50 a.m. We're off!

ME: It's a perfect day for travelling. Not too hot. Nice cool breeze.

BEN: Yeah. And it's supposed to warm up later.

ME: Oh goody.

BEN: What's making you smile?

ME: I'm rainbow spotting.

BEN: Has it rained?

ME: I'm looking out for drawings of rainbows displayed in windows – there's quite a few. All so beautifully different........ colourful and creatively lovely......... a symbol of hope.

BEN: I expect it makes a nice change to your old hobby –

ME: Umbrella spotting, yes.

BEN: The rainbow ones your favourite.

1.10 p.m.

ME: Feels *really really* good to be out of the house after almost twenty-four weeks. But some of the villages we've passed through have been a bit strange, like being in a science fiction movie – I didn't see a single soul. An it's sad to see the little village pubs closed.

BEN: Yeah.

ME: Think I'll have a bit of a lie-down now, after all the excitement of rainbow spotting and pretending I'm in a science fiction movie, like *The Village of the Damned*.

1.45 p.m.

BEN: Can you sit up for a moment and have a look to your left, there's gaps in the bushes.

ME: Beautiful! Seems a long time since I've seen rolling hills. A velvety patchwork quilt of soft greens, sewn together with lumpy, dark green wool. And there's a winding river.

BEN: Ooh, I hear a poem coming on.

ME: *Rainbows in windows*
*The wind in my hair*
*A winding river*
*And greens everywhere*

BEN: Very nice dear.

\* \* \* \* \* \* \* \*

2.15 p.m. We park in the car park next to the beach. I smile, breathing in the sea air.

ME: I'm glad there's no queue for the public toilets. I need to go again, had too many minty teas before we left..... Oops, my lace is untied.

*No queue for the loo*

317

*Lots of parking spaces too*
*Before I leave the car*
*Must tie lace on my shoe*

2.24 p.m.

ME:     It was good to see only one toilet cubicle was open. The rest had tape across them. There was a sign saying, one person at a time, markings on the floor showing where to walk in and out, and a man wearing a mask, sitting in what looked like a broom cupboard, keeping an eye on things. Seemed unreal. I was the only person there, and at first I stood there trying to make sense of all the tape and signs. Then the little man in the cupboard beckoned me in. I imagine there will be long queues on a hot, sunny weekend – so lucky me!

BEN:    Marvellous.

2.27 p.m.  We crunch our way along pebbles, Ben carrying a festival chair and the picnic cool box – men are so great at carrying things.

2.30 p.m.  I settled into my comfy festival chair (all the colours of the rainbow) at the top of the beach, by the beach front house gardens, while Ben went back to the car for his chair. I was pleased to see the bay was almost deserted, just a few couples and a family gathering – everyone social distancing.

* * * * * * * *

3.05 p.m.

ME:     It's getting warmer now the sun has come out.

318

BEN: Yeah (dozing with eyes closed after a hearty picnic).

ME: This is lovely, the sound of the waves and sea air. But do you know what I can see coming towards us from the horizon?

BEN: Dark storm clouds?

ME: No.

BEN: Pirates about to invade our shores?

ME: No.

BEN: A flock of hungry seagulls?

ME: Another big wave of pandemic approaching after the summer, followed by another lockdown before the end of the year. And more waves on the horizon after Christmas. And thousands more people dying and –

BEN: Try to think happy seaside thoughts dear. Sing a happy song.

ME: You're right.

*Oh, I do like to be beside the seaside*
*Oh, I do like to be beside the sea*

*And I would like to be under the sea, sea, sea*
*Where the octopuses sing*
*Squiddley de, de, de*

BEN: What are you like.

ME: It's lovely to see little children and hear their shrieks of joy as they splash about, excited in the shallows. There's a Labrador having great fun, galloping around like a little pony. And there's some baby seagulls over there. I've brought bread for the seagulls so I'll go and feed them when I've digested our delicious picnic.

BEN: You could sing to them too.

ME: *Oh, I do like to feed the little seagulls*
*And I do like to eat beside the sea*
*And I do like to throw lots of crumb, crumb, crumb*
*Helps to feed up many a hungry tum, tum, tum*

\* \* \* \* \* \* \* \*

4.25 p.m.

ME: Although it's a pebbly beach, now the tide is going out and lots of sand is appearing, it's nice to see children having fun, building their sandcastles.

BEN: Looks like it's dog-walk-before-dinner time too. More dogs have appeared.

ME: Must remember to bring a towel next time we go to the seaside, so I can have a little leap about in the water with the dogs.

BEN: For three seconds!

\* \* \* \* \* \* \* \*

ME: Remember our last boat trip to see the happy, wild seals at Seal Point, off the coast of Norfolk?...........

I forgot my reading glasses and just pointed the camera hopefully.

BEN:   And the photos came out really well!

ME:    Seems ages ago. I was enjoying myself so much, I didn't want to go back to dry land, just carry on out to sea, to distant shores, for adventures on remote islands.

BEN:   I didn't. I get sea sick.

* * * * * * * *

ME:    You've got lots of little black flies appearing on your jacket! Maybe it's because it's sandy coloured. They don't seem interested in my light blue hoodie with little boats and seagulls all over it.

BEN:   Oh yeah.

ME:    I wonder if they come from the garden behind us.

BEN:   What's that on your hand?

ME:    I don't know, I'll put me glasses on!..... Looks like a black ladybird with orange spots...... she's flown into my beach bag now, and landed on the cover of Celebrity Weekly, crawling on the Duchess of Cambridge's nose.

BEN:   A beach bug in a beach bag.

ME:    I'd better rescue her and put her in the garden behind us, she'll not want to come home with us.

BEN: I think I'll take a walk down the beach now.

ME: OK (gently lifting Celebrity Weekly out of beach bag).

4.33 p.m. I glanced up from perusing Celebrity Weekly, to see Ben waving at me from the sandy bit near the waters edge. Waves splashed onto his shoes. I waved back, smiling. Then blushed a little shell pink, as a family, quite a big family, sitting on the pebbles halfway between us, turned round to see who the man in the sandy coloured jacket, covered in flies, was waving at. They were a sea of little round curious faces. Mum, dad and lots of children.

4.34 p.m. I pretended to be *most awfully* interested in an article about Vanessa Feltz, who was talking about her recent weight loss. I feigned *great* admiration for her banana yellow top, strawberry red jeans and platform shoes – white with turquoise and yellow flower design. Very nice Vanessa!

4.35 p.m. I was *enthralled* by Katie Price, who informed readers that it wasn't her fault she'd been married so many times. Really Katie? And *delighted* to know Robbie Williams is reuniting with the band, Take That, for a special online performance for charity. Well done Robbie!

4.37 p.m. My eyes *lit up* when I turned the page to see that interior designer Kelly Hoppen had opened the doors to her stunning London home and shared her interior paradise secrets – black, white, silver and greys. Very elegant Kelly!

4.40 p.m. I didn't have to pretend to admire the page with rainbow design fashions – especially liked the white jumper with rainbow stripes and rainbow stick-on nails. The rainbow is a symbol of our times, and I think it would be nice if people wore it next 23$^{rd}$ of March, to celebrate our NHS and care workers – if they can afford rainbow fashions. Or wear rainbow face masks, if masks are still being worn. I've a feeling they will be.

5.05 p.m.    Ben crunched up the pebbly beach towards me, smiling a *revitalising-day-at-the-seaside* smile. I smiled back a *yes-wasn't-it* smile, noticing his jacket looked better.

ME:    There's no flies on you dear.

BEN:    Shall we head off soon?

ME:    Yes, getting chilly. It's been a lovely day beside the seaside (big yawn and stretch).

\* \* \* \* \* \* \* \*

7.04 p.m.    Home sweet home.

\* \* \* \* \* \* \* \*

*A sure cure for seasickness is to sit under a tree.*

Spike Milligan

**Almost five months later**

# November

8.21 a.m.

ME:      Day one of second lockdown!

BEN:     Yep.

ME:      You'll have to postpone visiting your sister. Hope Julia will be OK without the laptop you mended for her.

BEN:     I lent her my old one.

ME:      Oh, good.

BEN:     And we won't be able to take your dad out for a birthday meal.

ME:      Yes. It's a shame because he's housebound these days. But my sister texted the other day, to say she will be popping round to see him and ordering a takeaway pizza – he'll like that.

BEN:     He'll love the card I've ordered for him too.

ME:      Oh yes. The Dad's Army COVID Alert System card. It's hilarious. Tier **1** – photo of Hodges ordering someone to put their mask on. Tier **2** – Jones telling everyone not to panic. And Tier **3** – Frazer saying they're all doomed. Can't wait to see the card printed out!

BEN:     It'll arrive any day now.

ME:          Lovely! It'll make him laugh. And I'll use my paw print stamp to put paw prints on the envelope, that makes him smile too. And I'll write him a little letter.

* * * * * * * *

9.34 a.m.    I watch a single yellow leaf floating... down... down from the sycamore tree.... to gently... lay... down.... and lockdown into long rained-on-green grass.

9.35 a.m.    I sip dark green minty tea, slice and spread dark yellow banana onto toast, and smile as I remember reading, *Fairy Tale* (instead of Fair Trade) bananas and *Famous* (instead of Farmhouse) wholemeal bread on our Tesco shopping list.

9.36 a.m.    I enjoy fairytale banana on famous toast. Delicious.

I think the presenter on Radio Kent said we've just had the wettest October on record. Or did he say for years? A long time anyway.

9.37 a.m.    I wonder if it will be the coldest November on record (as I pull my dressing gown tighter around my shoulders). The wind felt icier when I fed the wildlife, first thing. My breath was a mist, billowing out in front of me, as if my brain fog was escaping out of my mouth.

*A leaf falls*
*From a tree*
*Am I moved*
*To poetry?*

*I don't know*
*Maybe*

9.44 a.m.

ME:    I wonder if there is a tree somewhere in the world, called a poe tree? Its branches swaying to its own rhythm. Its leaves falling to a waltz melody, only it can hear, in the circles of its mind.

*One two three*
*From the tree*
*One two three*
*From the tree*

BEN:    A poe tree in motion.

ME:    Yes!... Oh, I forgot to remind my sister, dad's birthday is coming up. Must text her before I forget.

BEN:    I forgot to turn the heating on. Getting chillier now.

ME:    *The weather's turning*
*So much colder*

BEN:    *And I'm feelin'*
*So much older*

ME:    *I pull my gown*
*Around my shoulder*

BEN:    *And you know*
*You should have told her*

I think you did tell her! You said she'd texted. You forgot that you remembered to remind her not to forget.

WE LAUGH

327

Is this really happening?

10.00 a.m.

BEN:      You look all *frowny*.

ME:       If restaurants and pubs are closed, I think the schools and colleges should be closed too.

BEN:      I agree.

ME:       I heard on Radio Kent, there was a rave, five hundred kids! The police had to break it up, and it got violent. Don't the police have enough to deal with? It's awful. Thoughtless individuals are going to be flouting the rules all over the place, with total disregard for others. I could hear the firework parties last night..... there were traffic jams...... and shops jam packed with shoppers, going crazy before lockdown. That's not going to help reduce the number of cases of the monster virus is it? And put even more pressure on our overworked NHS. And the nurses and doctors are getting ill and –

BEN:      Best take a break from listening to the radio and watching the news.

ME:       You're right. I'll tune into Classic FM. Heard one of Mozart's lovely symphonies the other morning. And some nice pieces by Brahms and Bach. Then Holst's *Mars* from *The Planets* was played – that energised me and got me out of bed!

BEN:      I'll get some composing done during this lockdown. Finish all the tunes I've been working on.

ME:       You'll get a musical *round-tuit*.

11.34 a.m.

BEN: Here's your Celebrity Weekly and Weekly Wife. Keep you quiet – I mean entertained for a while dear.

## Friday 6th

10.10 a.m.

BEN: We're booked up with slots for shopping until the sixteenth of November, so we're OK.

ME: That's great, well done you!

BEN: I got the slots before the internet got clogged up.

ME: I expect it started getting really busy as soon as the news of the lockdown came out.

BEN: Yeah. We've got a click and collect from Tesco on Monday. Here's the list if you want to add or delete anything.

ME: Lovely – gold star for you (reading list and cackling softly).

BEN: Got your M.E. eyeballs in again?

ME: I have. Guess what I read Ginsters Vegan Quorn Pasty as?

BEN: No idea. Can't wait to hear.

ME: Gangster's Vegan Quorn Patsy.

BEN: I don't like to imagine what gangsters would have in their pasties.

ME: Something nasty. Victim instead of vegan.

BEN: Do you still read *Fairy Tale* bananas instead of *Fair Trade* bananas? And Farmhouse bread as....

ME: *Famous* bread. Yes! And I'm still reading *Nightingale* Farm tomatoes as *Nightmare* Farm tomatoes and low fat *hummus* as low fat *humans*.

BEN: Maybe gangsters have low fat humans from nightmare farms in their pasties.

ME: You'll give me nightmares!

BEN: Sorry dear.

\* \* \* \* \* \* \* \*

1.00 p.m. I watch the news.

1.46 p.m. I comfort eat.

1.51 p.m. I write poetry.

2.01 p.m. I recite poetry to Ben.

*Is this really happening?*
*She said unto herself*
*As she found the honey jar*
*Sitting on the shelf*

*Is this really happening?*
*How are we to cope*

*All we can do, is do our best*
*We live, we pray, we hope*

*Is this really happening?*
*The sky is lockdown greys*
*We'll curl up cosy in our home*

BEN: *For twenty-something days!*

\* \* \* \* \* \* \* \* \*

2.03 p.m.

BEN: You must take a break from watching the news.

ME: I will. I *will try*. It's like trying not to watch *Coronation Street* when there's a very disturbing or upsetting storyline. You don't watch Monday or Wednesday's episodes, but by Friday, you *just have* to know what's happening! And if you miss a whole week, you end up feeling you've missed out on some good storylines that won't be enjoyable because you only got the tail end of the story, so you have no idea what's going on. And *who* is the new character? Why is she *so friendly* with Nick? And why is Sarah *so annoyed* with Alina? And why is Paul *so furious* with Todd? And you end up watching all the episodes you missed, in the omnibus at the weekend. And after you've watched it, you feel *so depressed,* you *swear* you won't do that again. But you do. Do you know what I mean?

BEN: Haven't a clue what you're talking about dear.

3.04 p.m.

ME: The four dear little saplings opposite our street have lost their leaves now. They look so young and slender, when I watch them swaying about, I find it hard to believe the strong winds we get up here haven't blown them over. I'm going to call them my poe trees.

BEN: You've been keeping an eye on them ever since they were planted haven't you.

ME: I have – the shrubs and the small lawn on the corner too! Have you noticed the shrubs are different, beautiful shades of green?

BEN: Can't say I have.

ME: It's been nice to see people come along to water them when they needed it in the summer. And it's been quite amusing when a man has stood with a big hose, squirting water with his back to me!

BEN: I'm sure it has.

ME: A builder left a huge plank of wood on the lawn, which annoyed me, and I'm sure must have really irritated the people taking care of it. Of course, when it was eventually removed, the grass had a long rectangular patch of yellow. But it can barely be seen now. No doubt the endless days of rain in October helped. Next time you peer out of the window or go out, have a look at it. It's lovely and green now.

BEN: Certainly dear.

ME:     The flats don't bother me anymore. The days have gone, when I watched them being built and would often think – *Is this really happening?* I listen to the radio and watch the news now and think –

BEN:    I know.

ME:     You know the teddy bears I've sat in the window, so that when people move into the flats, they won't see into our bedroom too well?

BEN:    Yeah. Di likes to sit between them and watch the world go by, twitching her whiskers.

ME:     I've seen little children looking up at them, so I make both teddies dance. You should see their sweet faces light-up!

BEN:    We'll be the house with the dancing teddy bears.

ME:     If you press their paws, they sing *Teddy Bear's Picnic* quite loudly. Very loudly really.

BEN:    I remember. I think our neighbours do too.

ME:     In the summer (giggling) I'll open the window, so the children can hear –

        *If you go down to the woods today*
        *You're sure of a big surprise*
        *If you go down to the woods today*
        *You'll never believe your eyes*

BEN:    *For every bear that ever there was*
        *Will gather there for certain because*

333

ME:     *Today's the day the teddy bears have*
        *Their picnic*

WE LAUGH

4.10 p.m.   I notice a tiny sycamore seed that has flown into our kitchen. It is on the floor next to the new addition to our family, who is curled up asleep, happily snoring on her special cushion. I stand, just smiling at her for a while. She is so lovely. Long grey fur. Cute grey nose and whiskers to match. Huge green eyes that make you melt like sunshine melting snow. And a big, contented I'm-so-happy-to-have-found-a-caring-home snore.

ME:     Cats are like chocolates, it's hard to have just one.

BEN:    Especially when they are as beautiful as Lovely.

4.11 p.m.   I pick up the sycamore seed and place it next to a sleeping fairy figurine in the window.

ME:     If we had an earthen floor, we get so many sycamore seeds flying into the kitchen this time of year, we'd have little trees growing.

BEN:    You'll have dreams of trees growing through the floorboards, now you've said that.

ME:     It'll make a nice change from dreaming about carnivorous COVID 19 monsters rampaging through hospitals and nurses wearing rainbow unicorns, I mean uniforms, running for their lives.

BEN:    You'll dream of unicorns with rainbow tails and manes, galloping through hospital corridors, now you've said that.

ME:      That would be nice...... I'd love to be shopping in America, in the supermarket where a shopper wears a unicorn costume – I saw it on *The Ellen DeGeneres Show*.

BEN:      I remember you saying..... You'd laugh so much, I'd be picking you up off the floor. Or you'd go up to it and pretend to feed it with asparagus tips.

ME:      True! And you'd be picking up old ladies who have fallen on the floor laughing at me.

BEN:      And little children would be asking mummy if they can feed the unicorn too.

ME:      There would be a queue to feed the unicorn, as well as at the checkouts!

\* \* \* \* \* \* \* \*

5.05 p.m.

ME:      In Celebrity Weekly, Claudia Winkleman says she has finally worked out what she wants in life. I wish she'd work out that the big shiny, black fringe that covers half her eyes doesn't suit her. If she wore a black face mask she'd look quite menacing, with all the black eyeliner she wears.

BEN:      Why does it bother you!?

ME:      No idea. Every time I see her on the ad for Head & Shoulders shampoo, on a game show, or a photo of her in one of my magazines, I get the urge to reach for my hair-cutting scissors and give her a good trim. There are seven photos of her in this article – Look!

BEN: See what you mean.

ME: I'll swear my right hand is starting to twitch.

BEN: Like when we've been out and you've seen youngsters with big, gaping holes in the knees of their jeans, and you *really* want to reach for a needle and thread.

ME: Their knees must get so cold at this time of year.

BEN: I quite agree (laughing).

ME: I'm looking forward to giving you another haircut. Your head is like my little sculpture. I like the shape of it – like a big white chocolate Easter egg.

BEN: Tasty looking and you'd hate to see me crack up!

ME: Yes (giggling). There's a photo of a very pretty face mask (turning the page of Celebrity Weekly) on the next page. It's black with a colourful red, yellow and orange flower design – Look.

BEN: Very floral.

ME: *Very expensive!*

BEN: Did you try on the new one I got you?

ME: Oh yes. I love the sky blue colour with white spots. And it's thin material, so I can breathe more easily than with the thick cotton one. I wonder if I wore a black one with orange spots, on Pevensey Bay beach, I'd attract the black ladybirds with orange spots we saw there. Like that time when we were in Devon, staying at your brother Dave's, and I wore leggings with a pale blue, lemon yellow and lilac, paisley design.

BEN: I remember.

ME: You remember? I'm amazed. It was almost thirty years ago!

BEN: We were sitting in the garden next to a bush with purple flowers, covered in butterflies.

ME: They were swallowtails, and I noticed the blue and yellow on their wings was the same as on my leggings. And the thin, black lines of the paisley design on my leggings was a little like the shape of some of the black lines on their wings. It was a buddleia bush, often known as the butterfly bush.

BEN: I remember your lap was covered in butterflies.

ME: It was *so delightful*. I felt like a mummy butterfly with her beautiful butterfly babies!

BEN: You've been a little flighty ever since.

WE LAUGH

ME: *Butterflies on the buddleia*
*Oh, what a pretty sight!*
*They rested on my leggings*
*Instead of taking flight*

Is this really happening?

*Happiness is a butterfly which, when pursued, is always beyond your grasp, but which, if you will sit down quietly, may alight upon you.*

Nathaniel Hawthorn

## Saturday 7th

11.03 a.m.    Ben returns home after his morning walk. He went into town today instead of by the river, and took some photos on his smartphone to show me. It was strange and a little spooky to see the high street deserted. Like when you see cities on the news during lockdown. I started to feel sad, but decided bursting into song was better than bursting into tears – a song by The Specials in the early eighties.

ME:    *This town is coming like a ghost town*
*All the clubs have closed down*
*This place is coming like ghost town*
*Bands won't play no more*

BEN:    The lyrics are very apt for these times.

ME:    Yes.

*Do you remember the good old days*
*Before the ghost town?*
*We danced and sang, and the music played*
*In the boomtown*

Do you know what?

BEN:    I'm not sure I want to hear. You've got that look in your eye.

ME:     You've taken lots of really good photos of our town, looking deserted, haven't you.

BEN:    Yeah.

ME:     Maybe you could make a short film using them, with *Ghost Town* as the sound track?

BEN:    That's a great idea!..... You sound very cheerful this morning.

ME:     I didn't listen to the news on Radio Kent first thing, or watch the news last night. And it's suddenly so chilly and quiet outside, it feels like Christmas Day.

BEN:    The kitchen cupboard and fridge looks Christmassy too, nicely stocked up after our delivery from Tesco.

ME:     That they do!

*  *  *  *  *  *  *  *

ME:     I've just been reading in –

BEN:    Celebrity Weekly?

ME:     Yes (giggling). Peter Andre's wife is going to put their Christmas decorations up early to make their little boy Theo's birthday full of festive cheer during lockdown, and Christmas seem longer. Emily says Lynda Bright –

BEN:    Who is that?

ME:     No idea, another celebrity I imagine. Anyway, Lynda has already put her tree up for her kids. Shall we put decorations up early? Emily says she doesn't care if it's supposed to be bad luck – Neither do I. Maybe put them up soon? Next week? (hesitant smile).

BEN: As early as you like dear.

ME: Goody! I'll make a start today.

*Drape gold tinsel here and there*
*It's November but I don't care*
*Then I'll flop into a chair*

BEN: *Gold lametta in your hair!*

I'll bring the snow globe down from the attic.

ME: Cool!... But not as icy cool looking as these photos in Celeb Weekly of a holiday destination in Finnish Lapland. I can *so imagine* wrapping up warm and riding on a sledge pulled by huskies through rows of snow-blanketed pine trees in this photo, look!

BEN: Very nice.

ME: The reindeer in this pic looks cuddly, I want to kiss his big hairy nose. And what a fine pair of antlers he has. You are encouraged to feed them a handful of reindeer moss – they prefer it to carrots apparently.

BEN: That's good to know.

ME: Can't you just see us cosy under blankets, riding on a sleigh pulled by reindeer.

BEN: Singing *Jingle Bells* (laughing).

ME: Of course! And there's places to stop off and drink hot berry juice, and eat freshly baked ginger cookies. And look at this beautiful photo of the setting sun, making the snowy scenery magical and sparkly – don't you just want to be there *right now!*

BEN: No, not really. After the stress of the journey and finding the accommodation isn't what was advertised, *and* there's hardly any vegetarian food, *and you* get upset because reindeer is on the menu, *and you* want to take a husky dog home with you because he looks *too old and tired* to be pulling a sledge and he takes a liking to you – we might wish we had stayed at home in the warm, instead of shivering in our boots with frozen toes. And *you do* catch a chill very easily, you're not getting any younger dear. You *do feel* the cold more than ever. You will need at least two cardies over your thermals and woolly jumper under a thick, heavy jacket. With all the weight you will hardly be able to move, which will make you fatigued. And cold air will make your asthma flare up.

ME: Thank you. That's my wonderful winter wonderland holiday daydream over!..... But you are right.

* * * * * * * * *

ME: There's some unusual Christmassy things in one of my catalogues today. Look at these gingerbread house tree decorations – so delightfully, intricately decorated.

BEN: Very sweet dear.

ME: And these glasses are amusing (pointing to frosted red and green baubles).

BEN:        They're Christmas tree baubles.

ME:         Look closer, they may look like decorations but they are the size of a tumbler, and there's a straw in the top!

BEN:        Oh yeah.

ME:         Aren't they fun!

BEN:        Great fun (yawning).

ME:         And these French liqueurs are nice – little bottles with labels, barrels and champagne corks. The corks make me cackle.

BEN:        That's good.

ME:         The wildlife advent calendars are nice, lets go mad and get two. One for now, one for next month! You could open some too. You're not usually bothered, but you'll enjoy it, every little picture is a surprise!

BEN:        Anything you say dear.

ME:         I think I'll get the dinky hedgehog tree decorations made out of straw for my niece who loves hedgehogs.

BEN:        Very rustic.

ME:         I'm most tempted by the floating candles.

BEN:        Don't we have them? The Led-lit tea lights that float in water?

ME:         These are more like white dinner candles that you suspend on clear acrylic string from the ceiling, and they are Led-lit. Look at the photo – they are like the floating candles in the Great Hall in the Harry Potter films.

BEN: Oh yeah, they do look good!

ME: Great for little kids who love the Harry Potter films.

BEN: And big kids.

DI: Meow! Meow! Hope you're going to give me a *Me-owee! Treat Stocking*, full of tasty cat biscuits, milky drops, a ball with a tinkly bell and sparkly balls to play with. But *no way* get me one of those Santa hats for cats that I've seen worn by tabby cats and kittens on your Christmas cards. And would you mind (big, endearing cat eyes), could you find it in your heart to decorate a Christmas tree for me to tear down the first day you put it up. It will be *so much more* fun than the gold tinsel snake or discarded Christmas wrapping paper – that I admit is good to hide under, roll about in or sit on, till it's nicely flattened. But the novelty soon wears off. I'd rather knock little novelties and tear baubles off tree branches, one by one, then rip off the tinsel and climb the tree so it comes crashing down into the fireplace, breaking the wings off your favourite glass angels – I'm *purring* at the thought.

ME: Of course we'll give you a cat stocking full of treats – but no tree this year I'm afraid. We gave it away to a charity.

BEN: But daddy will bring the snow lantern down from the attic. You love batting your paw on it to make the snow fall.

DI:   Oh yes. *Purrrrfect!*

LOVELY:   I've never had a Christmas cat stocking. Can I have one too?

ME:   Of course! You can have anything you desire.

LOVELY:   Can I have four calling birds, three French hens, two turtle doves, and a partridge in a pear tree?

\* \* \* \* \* \* \* \*

7.43 p.m.   Ben brings the musical snow lantern down from the attic, puts new batteries in, switches it on, and places it on top of the log burner. It lights up (twinkly lights sparkling in white tree branches).

7.45 p.m.   Diamanda leaps onto the coffee table, reaches her paw out and taps the lantern. Tiny, round, polystyrene snowflakes fall onto the top hats of snowmen (wearing red and green scarves) and music starts to play, sounding like a musical box. My miniature winter wonderland has come to life in the warmth of our home.

7.46 p.m.   Diamanda sits entranced in a satisfied cat way. We sing along to the music, as snow falls and golden flames dance in the log burner.

ME:   *Dashing through the snow*
*In a one horse open sleigh*
*O'er the fields we go*

BEN:   *Laughing all the way*

344

ME: *Bells on bob tails ring*
*Making spirits bright*
*What fun it is to laugh and sing*
*A sleighing song tonight*

BEN: *Oh, jingle bells, jingle bells*
*Jingle all the way*

ME: *Oh, what fun it is to ride*
*In a one horse open sleigh*
*Hey!*

Hey, are mince pies in the shops now? Did you get some?

BEN: I did! Fresh from Sainsbury's bakery.

ME: Ooh, hot mince pie with a glass of after dinner port?

BEN: Splendid idea.

8.16 p.m. I sneeze, which sets the snow lantern off again, down comes the snow, a new tune plays, and we burst into song.

ME: *We wish you a merry Christmas*
*We wish you a merry Christmas*
*And a happy New Year*

BEN: *Good tidings we bring to you and your king*
*We wish you a merry Christmas*
*And a happy New Year*

WE LAUGH

ME: Merry Christmas!

BEN:        Merry Christmas!

DI:         Meowy Christmas!

LOVELY:     Purry Christmas!

## Sunday 8th

8.36 a.m.

ME:         I've got it! I've got it!

BEN:        By jove she's got it! (Professor Higgins in *My Fair
            Lady* voice) What did you get dear?

ME:         The answer to a riddle I've just heard on the radio.
            See if you can get it.

            *I was called a man but never had a wife*
            *I was given a body but given no life*
            *I was given a mouth but given no breath*
            *Water gives me life but sun gives me death*

BEN:        I'm no good at riddles.

ME:         Have a think.

BEN:        Must I?

ME:         You must!

8.37 a.m.

BEN:        River?

ME: That's what I thought at first.

BEN: Give me a clue.

ME: My second idea was a snowflake.

BEN: A snowman!

ME: Yes!

## WE LAUGH

9.09 a.m.

ME: Do you know what storybook bear's birthday it is today?

BEN: Nope.

ME: Guess.

BEN: Must I?

ME: Yes.

BEN: Paddington Bear?

ME: No.

BEN: Pooh Bear?

ME: No, Rupert Bear. Remember him? With his red jumper, yellow check trousers and scarf to match?

BEN: Yeah.

ME:     He's one hundred years old today.

BEN:    Is he in a *care* bear *home* now?

ME:     The artist (giggling) who illustrated him, Mary Turtel, came from Canterbury. And there was a special wing dedicated to him in The Canterbury Heritage Museum. It closed a couple of years ago, so there's now a display in the Beaney House of Art and Knowledge.

BEN:    Would you like to visit there one day?

ME:     I would. And see the plaque in Ivy Lane where Mary Turtel spent her last years.... Rupert's clothes were originally a soft blue jumper and grey trousers. And he was a brown bear until The Daily Express cut inking expenses, giving him his iconic and characteristic white colour.

BEN:    Fascinating.

ME:     At the Beany House of Art and Knowledge there's also a display of *The Clangers*. Remember them, with the Soup Dragon?

BEN:    Yeah, they were amusing.

ME:     I was watching a vintage episode a few weeks ago. I love their woolly noses. And noticed that one of the planets in the background looked a lot like the coronavirus, shown in the background of the news readers on the news. Ugh.

BEN:    Not so amusing..... Do you like my new thick socks, for the wintery weather?

ME:      I like the soft blue colour, like Rupert's jumper used to be. And they look nice and woolly, like the Clanger's noses. Hope they'll fit OK inside your shoes.

> *I cannot feel amuse*
> *When I watch the news*
> *Do you think those thick socks*
> *Will fit inside your shoes?*

I wonder if the animators who made *The Clangers*, when they made a mistake, said they had dropped a clanger.

BEN:    You sound very cheerful again today!

ME:      Lots of things are making me smile. Firstly, I heard on Radio Kent about the new president in America, and was moved to write some verse, to be sung to the tune of *Nelly The Elephant*.

> *Oh Mr President*
> *Pack your trunk*
> *And trundle back*
> *To your circus*
> *Off you go with a*
> *Trumpety trump*
> *Trump! trump! trump!*

Secondly, our little stray is sleeping more and more indoors, instead of under the hedge, now the weather is chillier. She looks so contented, curled up in our warm kitchen, purring away when I stroke her. I think the name Lovely suits her.

BEN:    Yeah. She looks like a little grey bear, with her long, thick coat.

ME:     I've removed some of the fifteen horrible clumps of matted fur, but we'll have to ask the vet to do the rest, I'm afraid of cutting her skin.

BEN:    I'll take her soon. And will order a grooming brush and collar with a tag.

ME:     Can you get a pink collar with paw print design?

BEN:    Anything you say dear.

ME:     Thirdly, and best news of all. Your beautiful niece and her handsome hubby are recovering from the monster virus.

BEN:    Yeah, best news ever. Lets hope they make a complete recovery.

* * * * * * * *

10.35 p.m.  Ben returns home from his daily beneficial walk with an Autumn leaf stuck to his shoulder.

BEN:    That was refreshing! And there was no-one by the river.

ME:     Socks not too tight in your shoes then?

BEN:    Nope. Just right. And I took some photos to show you (getting his smartphone out of his pocket).

ME:     Oh, they are great! The sun on the trees and reflections in the river look so wonderfully Autumnal. What do you call a man under a pile of leaves?

BEN:    Dunno.

ME:        Russell.

BEN:      What do you call a man with a number plate on his head.

ME:        No idea.

BEN:      Reg.

ME:        What do you call a man with a very loud voice?

BEN:      Mike!

* * * * * * * *

11.00 a.m.  I open the back door and stand to attention in remembrance. Radio Kent has stopped playing music (just birdsong) and no-one is speaking for the two minutes silence.

11.02 a.m.

BEN:      Why are you standing there looking a little teary.

ME:        We were asked to stand at our front door for Remembrance Sunday, instead of going to commemorations. But I didn't want to stand at the front door.

BEN:      Bad hair day?

ME:        Yes.

BEN:      Bad face day?

ME:        Yes.

BEN:        Bad body day?

ME:         Yes – thanks for the compliments.

WE LAUGH

11.05 a.m.

ME:         Hot mince pie and coffee?

BEN:        Yeah (licking lips).

11.06 a.m.  Diamanda taps the snow lantern, snow starts to
            fall, the little music box plays another tune, and I
            sing along as I head for the kitchen.

ME:         *Chestnuts roasting on an open fire*
            *Jack Frost nipping at your nose*
            *La, la la la, la la la, la la la*

BEN:        *Merry Christmas tooo yooo!*

11.07 a.m.  I place two mince pies in the oven.

ME:         *Mince pies warming in the oven fire*
            *New socks fitting in your shoes*
            *La, la la la, la la la, la la la*

BEN:        *Merry Christmas with booze!*

11.08 a.m.  Ben gets his tool box from the cellar because he's
            going to get a *round-tuit* today.

BEN:        *Wing nuts, chisels and some bendy wire*
            *I'll get a round-tuit for you*

ME:        *You're doing this in the kitchen and the loo*

BEN:       *Merry Christmas tooo yooo!*

ME:        Did you know, a wing nut is an Asian tree that pro-
           duces characteristic broad-winged nutlets?

BEN:       Fascinating.

11.08 a.m. Diamanda curls up by the log burner.

ME:        *Cats love sleeping by an open fire*
           *Embers warm their ears and nose*
           *Whiskers and tails, and their furry bodies too*

BEN:       *Furry Christmas tooo yooo!*


## Monday 9th

8.26 a.m.  I draw a jolly Christmas tree and a snowflake with my
           fingertip in the condensation on the kitchen window,
           as my boiled eggs bubble away like excited children
           under the Christmas tree on Christmas morning. And
           my toast gets as toasty-hot as Santa's bum, hurtling
           down a chimney before the embers of a log fire have
           gone cold.

9.03 a.m.

ME:        Joan Collins and Mariah Carrey have put their Christ-
           mas trees and decorations up now (draping lamet-
           ta over fairy lights). I heard it on the radio. Vanessa
           Feltz said it's in the papers.

BEN:       Do you feel like a celebrity now you're putting up your decorations?

ME:      I am one! (huge celebrity grin). Can you give the house a hoover, Celebrity Weekly are popping round tomorrow to photograph us. I will have a bath and put on my *I'm-a-celebrity* makeup. And wear my life-is-*perfect*-and-I-have-a-lovely-man-and-two-*beautiful*-hairy-children-with-celebrity-names-and-don't-you-just-envy-my-*marvellous*-home smile. Then I'll find a couple of my best jumpers that haven't gone baggy and bobbly. And you'll need to smarten yourself up a bit – find something to wear that matches me a bit. Maybe wear that posh white shirt you don't like, with pleated panels down the front. You bought it to go with a posh, light charcoal grey three-piece suit for –

BEN:      A posh wedding I played at some archbishop's palace in Essex!

ME:      Yes (giggling), it will look good with me wearing my best Christmas jumpers – the grey one with a fluffy white polar bear, with black sequin eyes and the navy blue one with white snowflake design. Maybe the salmon pink one with cats all over it – I could pose with our hairy girls, wearing it. Lovely will look very posh with her Persian blue coat, and Diamanda's black coat is so shiny, she looks Polish. I mean polished. Do Polish people have shiny skins, I wonder? You worked with a nice Polish man, did he have a shiny complexion?

BEN:      No idea. But he did have a healthy glow!

ME:      I've already told Celebrity Weekly that I'm too tired to do more than one or two changes. They were very understanding because they've interviewed celebrities with M.E. – the actress Martine McCutcheon and yachtswoman Clare Francis. They'll interview me next week. I wonder what questions they will ask.... *How is breast feeding? Do you plan anymore children?*..... Oh sorry, that question is meant for Kelsey Parker..... *So you won't be going back to Los Angeles anytime soon?*...... Oops, that's a question for Gillian Anderson. *The scene where you cry in Ghost is so moving and realistic. How did you manage that?*..... Ah, that was yesterday's interview with Demi Moore. *How many years have you had M.E.?*....... Got it right this time!

WE LAUGH

I'll prepare myself by making some notes. My struggle for recognition as a writer. How I cope with the fame (giggling). How I keep sane in these difficult times. I'll be able to mention all the books I've written and the next one I'm writing, inspired by the film, *Rear Window*. It's an Alfred Hitchcock masterpiece of suspense, made in 1954. Have you seen it?

BEN:      Can't say I have.

ME:       It's about a photographer, played by James Stuart, who is stuck in a stuffy apartment during a heatwave, with a broken leg. Like us, the view out of his window is brick wall and lots of windows. He's so bored that he turns his zoom lens on his neighbours, and soon convinces himself that the chap across the way has murdered his wife. When the suspect realises he's being watched, our hero is in grave danger.... I've been observing a couple who have just moved in opposite, making notes for my book. And guess what happened the other day?

BEN:    Can't wait to hear.

ME:    The young man stared right up at me with dark, menacing, mixed race eyes, as he blethered into his mobile phone. So I've been spotted twice!

BEN:    Twice?

ME:    He saw me watching them moving in.

BEN:    Are you in grave danger now?

ME:    Yes, isn't it exciting!

WE LAUGH

ME:    Would you like to hear some of my notes?

BEN:    I must reply to some e-mails and texts but I'm sure you are going to tell me. I'm all ears.

ME:    The first thing I noticed was the delivery van with *Fantastic Removals* written on the side. There was also a photo of two, smiling, British, clean shaven, handsome young men in their twenties, carrying boxes – looking *fantastically helpful*. When the delivery men emerged from the van, I noticed they were two, ugly, grumpy, beardy men. One looked in his fifties, the other in his thirties. Both looked and sounded *very unhelpful*. And Italian.

BEN:    So nothing like advertised!.... I saw them. One was taking a break with a fag, and when he'd finished –

ME: Threw it on the shrubs..... Anyway, the first thing I saw carried out of the van by Mr Grumpy the elder, was a shiny, metal pedal bin. Then Mr Grumpy the younger carried a pretty floral patterned ironing board and a white, rattan laundry basket – same as our new one. So we have something in common with our new neighbours!

BEN: That's nice.

ME: A small, plump, young Indian woman and her tall, slim partner, who looked like Mr Bored and Sulky, heaved bulging carrier bags out of the boot of a dark blue SEAT Leon. She looked like Mrs Tired and Stressed as she lifted red M&S bags and white Primark bags. They shop more at Primark than M&S, I think. The bigger bags were Primark.

BEN: Very observant dear. I'll award you a nosey neighbour of the year award.

ME: Will I get an engraved resin or golden sculpture of a house, with a little person staring out of the window?

BEN: Yeah.

ME: Lovely!.... Anyway, next to appear from the van was was a huge plasma TV and lots of flat-packs. I can see the woman now, in my mind's eye, slaving over a pretty floral ironing board, next to piles of clean washing. Picking up his dirty laundry and stuffing it into the white laundry basket. And throwing rubbish into the shiny metal bin that's overflowing, because he never empties it and she's hoping he will take the hint. But he's too busy –

BEN:      Lounging on a sofa.

ME:       A leather sofa.

BEN:      How do you know it's a leather sofa, did you see it?

ME:       No, but he looks a leather-sofa-internet-surfer type. The sofa will be arriving at a later date. My witchy senses tell me.

BEN:      He'll lounge and watch sport on his huge plasma TV, with a can of beer, biriani and onion bhajis.

ME:       He looks athletic and goes to the gym. I saw him carry a black holdall with Adidas written on the side.

BEN:      He'll probably be sulky because the gyms are closed for the lockdown.

ME:       And she'll be tired and stressed because she works for the NHS.

BEN:      How do you know, witchy senses again?

ME:       No, some clothes fell out of one of her bulging carrier bags, and I thought I saw a nurse's uniform. And he drinks a lot of water. He carried packs of bottles wrapped in plastic from the car. One pack split open and a bottle fell out. It rolled across the road and under your car. I wondered if he'd crawl under your car to get it.

BEN:      And did he?

ME:       He didn't need to, it rolled under to the edge of the kerb. He strode across the road without looking to see if any traffic was coming and almost –

BEN:     Got flattened like a flat-pack.

ME:      Yes. When he retrieved the bottle he was right out-side our front room window. And I got a close look.

BEN:     Did you tap on the window and give him a little wave? (laughing).

ME:      No, but he saw me watching and scowled. I re-named him Mr Sulky with an air of Aggression and a neck full of tattoos, and wanted to inform him that he'd regret all the white furniture that I'd just seen carried out of the van by Mr Grumpy senior. Or rather, Mrs Tired and Stressed would regret it. Espe-cially if they got a pet or had kids. The Morrisons van that nearly ran him over, parked *on the bright side of the road*, and the delivery man was whistling *Brown Eyed Girl*. So I named him Mr Van Morrison.

BEN:     What are you like.

ME:      A very nosey neighbour who calls people names for a bit of fun.... Oh, and I wanted to mention to Mr Sulky that they'd never fit a week's worth of all his tall man clothes and her short, very wide clothes into the white rattan laundry basket. It's so much smaller than it looked in the catalogue and is quite flimsy – we know because we have one the same. We don't use it but our cat likes to scratch it, hide under a bath towel if you drape it over the basket, or curl up on top of it, especially if you've just put a little pile of clean, warm towels on top, ready for bath time.

BEN:        I expect Mrs Tired and Stressed will tell him.

ME:          If they are talking to each other after she shrunk some of his favourite, expensive Adidas tee-shirts because she accidentally put them on a very hot wash, after a tiring stressful day at the hospital. And he is putting on weight during lockdown, so the tee-shirts are extra tight, because she wants to impress him by feeding him lots of delicious, spicy, oily, Indian cuisine, with mountains of naan bread.

BEN:        This will make him even more sulky.

ME:          The last of the delivery was lots of small boxes. They didn't look labelled. So when Mrs Tired and Stressed disappeared into the front of the flat, and he just paced about as if marking his territory, or leaned out of an open window, peering up and down our street, I imagined she was sorting through the boxes in an effort to find plates so they could eat dinner. It was late in the day and they were both hungry because there wasn't time for lunch... She gets tired and gives up looking because she needs the energy to make the bed. He just wants to set up the TV to watch *Men Behaving Badly* with a take-away pizza in a box. But she'd rather watch *The Good Karma Hospital* with a good, creamy korma.

BEN:        So, in your book, who will murder whom?

ME:          I haven't decided. Maybe she'll have an affair with the Morrisons delivery man, because he sings *Brown Eyed Girl* to her with twinkly Irish eyes and makes her giggle like a schoolgirl. And because she's tired of working long hours at the hospital, and the staff are over-worked, constantly cleaning because of the

COVID-19 virus, and constantly fear they may get it because it's *so contagious*. Then she comes home and has to constantly clean white surfaces and wash clothes and iron on her pretty floral ironing board, that no-longer seems pretty, and take constant criticism of her cooking skills and cope with his laziness and dominating the TV viewing *and* she's always trying to stuff clothes that need washing into the tiny, white rattan laundry basket, and stuff rubbish into the small, shiny metal pedal bin, while he stuffs his face with pizza, but blames her cooking for his weight gain.

One day Mr Sulky with an air of Aggression, finds her in bed with Mr Van Morrison. He had been wondering why so many treats had been delivered free of charge. Tasty sweet and savoury pastries. Chocolate cake and chocolate biscuits..... So he'll plan to kill her and make it look like suicide because she feels guilt.

She has a feeling he is planning something bad and makes her own plans to run off with Mr Van Morrison. But she'll catch the COVID virus at the hospital where she works. And after a long battle with the illness. Will die. Then he'll be Mr Sad, Sulky and Sorry-for-himself because he has to look after himself, and realises he took her for granted and was often thoughtless and cruel. And be full of remorse and drink a lot, far too much, and one day step out into the road, trying to retrieve shopping that's fallen out of his bag, into the road, and be knocked down by a Morrisons delivery van.

And when my play is on Radio 2, they'll play Van Morrison singing *Brown Eyed Girl*. And they'll play

Is this really happening?

him singing *The Bright Side Of The Road* too, because that's where the delivery man used to park his
Morrisons van on a sunny afternoon.

WE LAUGH

Anyway, back to the interview with Celeb Weekly.
I'll mention all the groovy music you've composed.
And you could pose, looking creatively thoughtful
with your guitar, wearing the black shirt I gave you
with musical notes all over it, or the white one with
black musical notes all over it. You'd look nice wearing your posh, light charcoal grey three-piece suit,
with Lovely and her long, grey, posh looking fur, on
your lap.

BEN:    I'm *relieved* this is all in your imagination dear. And
        have you been drinking my *real* coffee again?

ME:     I may have had one..... Or two. Goes magnificently
        with a mince pie..... Or two.

11.32 a.m.

ME:     We got a couple of nice letters from my penpals
        Shauna and Jim. Want to read them?

BEN:    I'm just nipping into town, I'll read 'em later. Are
        they doing OK?

ME:     Yes, keeping busy. And Jim sent another of his lovely
        poems you'll like, and one written by his little grand-
        son – only five years old. It's delightful! Jim says he's
        a poetic chip off the grandpa block. And he's right.
        I'll read them to you later.

362

BEN: Want anything from Sainsbury's?

ME: More mince pies please.

12.47 p.m.

ME: With your birthday cards still up, and Shauna and Jim's cards, *and* the Christmas decorations, it looks like it's close to Christmas already doesn't it? I think I'll watch the film premiere of *It's Beginning To Look A Lot Like Christmas*. It's on this afternoon.

BEN: Oh no (hand on head), I think I can hear some singing coming on.

ME: Maybe!....... Do you fancy feeling more Christmassy with a coffee and hot mince pie?

BEN: Yeah!

ME: *It's beginning to look a lot like Christmas*
*Everywhere you go*
*Take a look in the Five and Ten*
*Glistening once again*
*With candy canes and silver lanes aglow*

*It's beginning to look a lot like Christmas*
*Toys in every store*
*But the prettiest sight to see*
*Is the holly that will be on your own front door*

\* \* \* \* \* \* \* \*

ME: Nothing like a hot mince pie with a nice hot cuppa on a cold winter's day.

BEN: I quite agree dear. Do you feel some verse coming on?

ME: *There's nothing like a hot mince pie*
*Warms you to your heart*

BEN: *There's nothing like Brussels sprouts*
*Make you want to –*

ME: What are you like.... I found two old crackers in the Christmas decorations box – lets go mad and pull them!

BEN: OK.

### CRACK!

ME: Hurrah, I got a purple crown, joke and wee gift – a sweet miniature pack of cards. What do you get when you cross Santa with a duck?

BEN: Dunno, what do you get when you cross Santa with a duck?

ME: A Christmas quacker.

BEN: Not the best of cracker jokes.

ME: I know a couple of good ones. Well, I like them. What carol is heard in the desert?...... Oh camel ye faithful!

BEN: Not bad.

ME: Why is it getting harder to buy Advent calendars?..... Because their days are numbered..... Lets pull another cracker.

### CRACK!

ME: Hurrah! I got the prizes again. But I'll let you have them.

BEN: I'm thrilled. Green paper crown and a black, plastic moustache. Just what I always wanted.

ME: The moustache will make you look like Hercule Poirot. You could do your impression of him!

BEN: Mon ami *Hashtings* (holding plastic moustache in place with upper lip).

ME: Brilliant (cackling).

BEN: What do you call an old snowman?

ME: I don't know, what do you call an old snowman?

BEN: Water.

ME: That's a good one!

BEN: I know one. When is a boat like snow?..... When it's adrift.

ME: Let's put the paper crowns on! (smiling).

BEN: Anything you say dear.

* * * * * * * *

ME: I had a funny dream last night.

BEN: Funny? Not the usual weird disturbing dreams or nightmares?

ME: Yes, for a pleasant change. You know that programme I've started to watch. The one that's a bit like *Gogglebox,* but it's couples who've been on *90 Day Fiancé,* watching footage of other couples on *90 Day Fiancé,* and commenting?

BEN: *Four In A Bed?*

ME: No, there's only two on a bed in the programme – *Pillow Talk.....* What was I talking about?

BEN: The funny dream.

ME: Oh yes. The couples commenting on other couples.

BEN: Were they commenting on you?

ME: No, but ooh, what a horrible thought! I can imagine them saying – *Look at the state of her hair...... She needs to wear some makeup...... Not very fashion conscious is she....... Watches far too much TV..... Plods about like an old person......... Thinks about chocolate too much...... Thinks too much.*

BEN: *Dreadful singing voice.... Annoying cackle.... Very nosey neighbour.*

ME: Thank you for that dear. Anyway, do you want to hear my dream? Bit of a long story.

BEN: I'm sure it will be most amusing.

ME: The dream started with me peering out of the bedroom window.

BEN: Being a nosey neighbour.

ME:     Of course! And I noticed all the couples in *Pillow Talk* were gathered outside our house, pointing to the flats opposite and commenting. Then one of our regional news reporters appeared, standing at a distance, wearing a mask and started telling them the latest news about people moving into the flats. We decided to join them and could hear everyone whispering, 'Is this really happening?' And it was a bit creepy because as we mingled and tried to speak to them, we realised we were invisible. Then all the couples and families in our street started to step out of their front doors, onto the path, whispering about the pandemic and the new housing estate – *Is this really happening? Is this really happening?*

BEN:    Spooky.

ME:     Everyone was wearing masks with different animal prints – tiger, leopard, giraffe and snakeskin. Tony from *Time Team* appeared wearing a skull mask and his team of archaeologists wore dinosaur masks. Then it all got a little crazy.

BEN:    Sounds good.

ME:     All the neighbours in our street, couples from the TV programme and Tony's time team, started galloping about happily making animal noises. Those wearing snakeskin masks wriggled playfully on the path. Children, wearing dog and bunny masks, barked and hopped about.

BEN:    What did Tony do?

ME:     He danced, with his teeth chattering behind a skull

367

mask. Then four calling birds, three French hens and two turtle doves appeared flying around their heads.

BEN: Was there a partridge in a pear tree?

ME: There was a partridge perching in one of the saplings.

BEN: Did you burst into song?

ME: I did, and you laughed your Christmas socks off. And everyone lived, barking madly and hoppily, happily ever after. *THE END.*

Oh! Nearly forgot. Want to hear Jim's poems?

BEN: Yeah!

ME: The poem he wrote is entitled Inspiration.

*I love your little poems*
*They go straight to my heart*
*Inspiring my poetic muse*
*But where am I to start?*

*First think up a theme*
*That's easy as can be*
*I'll write about seashells*
*Or beasties in the sea.*

*The tomatoes in the greenhouse*
*Or maybe purple peas*
*The snails in the garden*
*Or the birdies in the trees.*

*There must be lots of poems*
*So much that I can say*

*But my muse is quite exhausted*
*I'll leave it for another day.*

BEN:  Excellent!

ME:  Yes, *but wait* until you hear some verse by his little grandson, Eddie.

*Wood is important*
*Food is important*
*Pirates like pitta bread*
*Monkeys like monkey bananas*
*The End*
*not quite*
*Actually that is not*
*the real end*
*Whales like water*
*The Real End*

BEN:  Brilliant!

ME:  How does Christmas Day end?

BEN:  With us relieved to get home?

ME:  It ends with the letter Y.


**THE REAL END**

Is this really happening?

*Learn from yesterday, live for today, hope for tomorrow.*

Albert Einstein